SELF-ASSESSMENT

IN

CHEST MEDICINE

SELF-ASSESSMENT
IN
CHEST MEDICINE

▼

Ronald B. George, M.D.

Professor and Chairman

Department of Medicine

Louisiana State University School of Medicine

Shreveport, Louisiana

Michael A. Matthay, M.D.

Professor of Medicine and Anesthesia

Associate Director, Intensive Care Unit

Senior Member, Cardiovascular Research
   Institute

School of Medicine

University of California, San Francisco

San Francisco, California

Richard W. Light, M.D.

Professor of Medicine

University of California, Irvine

Veterans Administration Medical Center

Long Beach, California

Richard A. Matthay, M.D.

Boehringer Ingelheim Professor of Medicine

Associate Chairman

Pulmonary and Critical Care Section

Yale University School of Medicine

New Haven, Connecticut

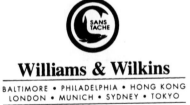

Williams & Wilkins

BALTIMORE • PHILADELPHIA • HONG KONG
LONDON • MUNICH • SYDNEY • TOKYO

A WAVERLY COMPANY

Editor: Kathleen Courtney Millet
Production Coordinator: Kimberly S. Nawrozki
Copy Editor: Michaelann Zimmerman, Shelley C. Potler
Designer: Dan Pfisterer
Typesetter: Peirce Graphic Services, Inc.
Printer: Victor Graphics

Copyright © 1996
Williams & Wilkins
351 West Camden Street
Baltimore, Maryland 21201–2436 USA

Accurate indications, adverse reactions, and dosage schedules for drugs are provided in this book, but it is possible that they may change. The reader is urged to review the package information data of the manufacturers of the medications mentioned.

Printed in the United States of America

Library of Congress Cataloging in Publication Data

Self-assessment in chest medicine / Ronald B. George . . . [et al.].
    p.   cm.
    Companion volume to: Chest medicine / edited by Ronald B. George . . . [et al.]. 3rd ed. c1995.
    ISBN 0-683-03460-X
    1. Chest—Diseases—Examinations, questions, etc. 2. Respiratory intensive care—Examinations, questions, etc. I. George, Ronald B.
    [DNLM: 1. Lung Diseases—examination questions. 2. Lung—physiology—examination questions. 3. Critical Care—examination questions. WF 18.2 S465 199]
    RC941.C5675 1995 Suppl.
    616.2'4'0076—dc20
    DNLM/DLC
    for Library of Congress   95-35114
                                             CIP

95 96 97 98 99
1 2 3 4 5 6 7 8 9 10

Reprints of chapter(s) may be purchased from Williams & Wilkins in quantities of 100 or more. Call Isabella Wise in the Special Sales Department, (800) 358-3585.

Preface

Medicine continues to change rapidly, and new information appears regularly. The American Board of Internal Medicine has made the decision that all certification will be time limited in the future, meaning that physicians will be continually tested for knowledge of the latest advances. For the busy practicing physician and the harried trainee, keeping abreast of the latest information is a constant challenge. Self-assessment during home study is probably the most common method by which this important task is accomplished.

Self-Assessment in Chest Medicine is designed as a companion to the Third Edition of *Chest Medicine.* While self-assessment supplements are available for several popular medical texts, none has yet been produced to accompany a textbook of pulmonary and critical care medicine. This review book is designed for use by house staff physicians, fellows, practicing physicians, and allied health specialists in the area of pulmonary and critical care medicine, and for general internists and family physicians who wish to update their knowledge in these areas. It is priced so that physicians in training can readily obtain it for home use, and it is designed so that brief study periods may be used productively.

The questions are designed to be pertinent, but not confusing or necessarily hard. We have attempted to avoid trick questions or double meanings. All questions are based upon the material contained in the Third Edition of *Chest Medicine.* They are arranged by chapter, with answers and discussion falling at the end of each chapter. Each question has been reviewed by the editors, several clinicians, and outside reviewers.

To keep down the costs of the review book, we have not reproduced illustrations from the textbook, nor have we duplicated references. Current bibliographies are contained in each of the textbook chapters, to which the reader is referred for more detailed review of the subject matter. The appropriate pages of the textbook are cited at the end of each discussion.

We would like to thank those individuals who worked hard and rapidly to make this review book available in time for board review. In particular, we would like to express our thanks to Jeff McCartney, M.D., who came up with the idea for this book, and the other contributors at Louisiana State University School of Medicine, University of California, San Fransisco, and Yale University School of Medicine, who did the major work of creating the questions. For overseeing the expeditious publication of the review book we wish to thank Katey Millet, as well as the other editors and proofreaders at Williams & Wilkins.

Ronald B. George, M.D.

Richard W. Light, M.D.

Michael A. Matthay, M.D.

Richard A. Matthay, M.D.

Contents

Pulmonary Structure
and Function

chapter 1

Functional Anatomy of the Respiratory System

QUESTIONS

Question 1.1. **A 20-year-old man sustains a basilar skull fracture in an automobile accident. The patient has some accessory muscle use; however, he is unable to maintain adequate ventilation and requires intubation and mechanical ventilation. Which of the following statements is/are true?**

A. The medullary center and the rostral pontine respiratory nuclei are likely involved in this patient's injury.
B. The ventral respiratory group of the medulla containing both inspiratory and expiratory nuclei is likely continuing to function despite the injury.
C. The dorsal respiratory group is functioning normally as manifest by the accessory muscle use.
D. Normal voluntary control of respiration is governed primarily by the brainstem.
E. Intrinsic automaticity of respiration is regulated by both the ventral and dorsal respiratory groups.

Question 1.2. **Regarding cortical modulation and the mechanoreceptors of respiration, which of the following is/are true statements?**

A. Voluntary respiratory pathways originate in cortical neurons with efferent projections, via corticospinal and corticobulbar pathways, to respiratory associated muscles.
B. There are three kinds of pulmonary parenchymal receptors in the lung that send afferent signals to the CNS via the corticospinal nerves.
C. The Hering-Breuer reflex may produce apnea by stimulation of the juxtacapillary receptors within the interstitial spaces of the lungs.
D. The activity of the expiratory muscles may increase by exciting the stretch receptors.
E. The receptors felt responsible for mediating the rapid, shallow breathing characteristic of interstitial edema and interstitial fibrosis are the juxtacapillary receptors.

Question 1.3. **Which of the following are true statements concerning the effects of changes of $PaCO_2$ and PaO_2 on the respiratory drive?**

A. Lack of oxygen is the most important chemical stimulus in the regulation of respiration in normal individuals.
B. Most of the increase in minute ventilation is in response to changes in the oxygen concentration in the cerebrospinal fluid.
C. The effect of hypercarbia on increasing ventilation is by stimulation of the peripheral chemoreceptors located in the carotid and aortic bodies.

3

D. Unlike the central stimulating effect of hypercarbia, the central effect of hypoxia is respiratory depression.

E. A low pH at a constant $PaCO_2$ can result in increased minute ventilation.

Question 1.4.   Which of the following is/are correct regarding the structures of the pharynx, larynx, and trachea?

A. A right vocal cord injury is possible with surgery of the aortic arch.

B. Bilateral vocal cord paralysis causes a variable extra thoracic airway obstruction.

C. Bilateral vocal cord paralysis produces an expiratory stridor.

D. In the unconscious patient, the head should be hyperextended and the jaw pulled forward to maintain airway patency.

E. Normally the respiratory tract is free of bacteria below the level of the larynx.

Question 1.5.   Regarding the gas exchange area of the alveoli and associated structures, which of the following is/are true?

A. Interlobular septa contain lymphatic channels which when distended by fluid are manifest as Kerley's "B" lines.

B. Most of the alveolar surface is covered by the Type I cells, and when injured they are unable to replicate.

C. Type II granular pneumocytes differentiate into Type I cells after injury to restore the gas exchanging alveolar surface.

D. Surfactant secretion is increased by cholinergic but not adrenergic stimulation.

E. Type I cells are responsible for surfactant production.

Question 1.6.   Several clearance and defense mechanisms exist within the lungs. Select the true statement(s) regarding these mechanisms.

A. Particle sizes of 10 micrometers in diameter or smaller are routinely deposited in the terminal bronchioles but not the alveoli.

B. Ninety percent of the particles directly deposited on the mucus layer are cleared within 2 hours in the normal lung.

C. Alveolar macrophages originate in the bone marrow and subsequently adapt for the aerobic environment of the lungs.

D. Cytokines and chemotactic factors such as leukotriene B_4 and interleukin-8 are derived from the Type II pneumocytes.

E. Alveolar macrophages gain entry into regional lymph nodes by exiting the alveolar interstitial space into the adjacent lymphohematogenous system.

Question 1.7.   The lungs are richly supplied with lymphatic vessels. Select the true statement(s) that most closely describe their anatomy and function.

A. Two purposes of the pulmonary lymphatics are to keep the alveoli clear of excess fluid and to serve as channels for macrophages to migrate to regional lymph nodes.

B. In general, the upper lobes drain into the subcranial lymph nodes.

C. Airway lymphocytes are thought to participate in local responses to antigens with both a local and generalized production of immunoglobulins, particularly IgE.

D. Movement of lymph is increased by respiratory movements coupled with a series of valves in the lymphatic vessels.

Question 1.8.   A 47-year-old man sustains bilateral phrenic nerve injuries after surgery in the mediastinum. Which statement is correct regarding this patient?

A. Resting tidal volume depends on the muscles of inspiration and will be no different from baseline in this patient.

B. Elevation and increases in the diameter of the lower rib cage will continue to function via normal mechanisms.
C. Sensory innervation of the costal portion of the diaphragm will be unaffected.
D. The internal intercostal muscles will be recruited to a greater extent to aid with inspiration.

Question 1.9. **A 30-year-old man sustains a knife injury to the right hilum. Prior to repair of the injury, the physician may consider which one of the following to be true?**

A. Blood supply to the right lung would be compromised only to the level of the segmental bronchi by severing the bronchial artery.
B. Nutritive blood supply to the lung is adequate if the right bronchial artery is intact.
C. Major bronchial arteries to each lung originate from the aorta and the ipsilateral brachiocephalic artery.
D. The physician can expect a right to left shunt of up to 5% of the cardiac output to be present under normal circumstances.

Question 1.10. **Match the following cells and structures of the lungs (A through F) with their appropriate numbered description. Answers are used only once.**

A. Serous cells
B. Mucus cells
C. Clara cells
D. Kulchitsky cells
E. Pores of Kohn
F. Canals of Lambert

1. Progenitors for ciliated cells, brush cells, and goblet cells
2. Holes that connect alveoli directly
3. Hypertrophy of is a measurement in the Reid index
4. Secrete a variety of peptides including lysozyme, lactoferrin, and the secretory leukoprotease inhibitor
5. Passages from distal airways to adjacent alveoli
6. Cells common to newborns and may be precursors of bronchial carcinoid tumors and small cell carcinomas

ANSWERS

Answer 1.1. **A, B, E - True; C, D - False**

The control of breathing is governed by the interplay of cortical and brainstem respiratory pathways. The medullary center appears to be the generator of respiratory rhythm, while groups of rostral pontine respiratory nuclei seem to act to "fine tune" respiratory regulation. Two areas of the medulla, the dorsal respiratory group (DRG) and the ventral respiratory group (VRG), control autonomic respirations. Any override of intrinsic automaticity involves the cortex. The VRG contains inspiratory and expiratory bulbospinal neurons whose output is to the spinal respiratory motor neurons for intercostal, abdominal, and phrenic innervation and auxiliary muscles of respiration. The DRG is composed of inspiratory bulbospinal neurons providing input to the spinal inspiratory neurons of the phrenic and external intercostal nerves.

Reference: pages 4, 5

Answer 1.2.   **A, D, E - True; B, C - False**

Pathways of voluntary maneuvers such as coughing, singing, and speaking originate in the cortex which sends out efferent projections to the respiratory associated muscles via the corticospinal and corticobulbar pathways. Several receptors have been identified in the lungs and their associated muscles of respiration which send signals back to the CNS via the vagus nerve. Lung inflation may initiate apnea (Hering-Breuer reflex) by stimulation of the stretch receptors, thus increasing the activity of the expiratory muscles. The juxtacapillary receptors are within the interstitium of the alveolar wall and may mediate the rapid, shallow breathing seen in interstitial fibrosis and interstitial edema.

Reference: pages 5, 6

Answer 1.3.   **D, E - True; A, B, C - False**

Carbon dioxide is the most important chemical stimulus in the regulation of respiration in normal individuals. The central nervous system (CNS) is sensitive to elevations in $PaCO_2$, and thus hydrogen ion concentration, as a stimulus to increase minute ventilation. The peripheral chemoreceptors, carotid and aortic bodies, are sensitive to reductions in PaO_2 and increase minute ventilation by an alternate mechanism. Paradoxically, hypoxia in the CNS induces respiratory depression while CNS hypercarbia will increase minute ventilation. A low pH at a constant $PaCO_2$ can result in an increased minute ventilation.

Reference: page 6

Answer 1.4.   **B, D, E - True; A, C - False**

Vocal cord injuries are further manifestations of some intrathoracic diseases or surgical procedures. The left recurrent laryngeal nerve descends under the aortic arch and therefore any mediastinal mass, tumor, or surgical manipulation in the area may subsequently affect the left vocal cord. Bilateral vocal cord paralysis causes a variable extra thoracic airway obstruction and produces an inspiratory stridor. To maintain airway patency in an unconscious patient, the head should be hyperextended and the jaw pulled forward. The lungs and trachea are normally free of any bacteria.

Reference: pages 11, 12

Answer 1.5.   **A, B, C - True; D, E - False**

Five major cell types have been identified in the alveoli of the lungs (Type I cells, Type II cells, endothelial cells, interstitial cells, and macrophages). Endothelial cells account for about 30% of the cells in the human lung parenchyma. The Type I alveolar lining cells participate in gas-exchange and if injured cannot replicate. The Type II granular pneumocytes differentiate into Type I cells allowing for restoration of the gas exchanging surface. Interlobular septa are spaces between pulmonary lobules and when filled with fluid or fibrosis are manifest as Kerley's "B" lines. Surfactant secretion is by cholinergic, adrenergic, and hyperventilation stimulation. Secretion of surfactant is by the Type II granular pneumocytes.

Reference: pages 16, 17

Answer 1.6.   **B, C, E - True; A, D - False**

Lung clearance and defense mechanisms include the mucociliary escalator, alveolar macrophages, and lymphohematogenous drainage. Particle sizes of 10 micrometers or greater are directly deposited in the upper respiratory passages, while those below 10 micrometers are carried into the distal respiratory tract. Ninety percent of the particles directly deposited on the mucus layer are cleared within 2 hours. Alveolar macrophages originate in the bone marrow and initially circulate as monocytes. Eventually the monocytes adapt to their aerobic environment in the lungs. The alveolar macrophages are responsible for cytokine production and the recruitment and activation of other inflammatory cells through macrophage-derived chemotactic factors. Once phagocytosis has occurred, the macrophages may exit the interstitium and enter the lymphohematogenous system to migrate to regional lymph nodes where they may reside indefinitely.

Reference: pages 18–21

Answer 1.7.   **A, D - True; B, C - False**

The lymphatics of the lungs serve to remove fluid from the interstitial spaces and participate in the alveolar defense mechanism by transporting macrophages from distal areas of the lungs. The distribution of lymphatic drainage varies somewhat; however in general, the lower lobes drain into the hilar and subcarinal nodes, while the upper lobes more often drain directly to the paratracheal nodes. The mucosal immunity is intact largely because of airway lymphocytes which initiate local responses to antigen and immunoglobulin production, particularly IgA. Lymph moves through the vessels as a result of respiratory movements coupled with a series of one-way valves in the lymphatic vessels.

Reference: page 21

Answer 1.8.   **C**

Phrenic nerve paralysis is manifested by the loss of diaphragm function during inspiration. The diaphragm, a muscle of inspiration like the external intercostals and the parasternal intercartilaginous muscles, is responsible for resting tidal volume. Recruitment of other muscles of inspiration would be necessary to maintain tidal volume in the resting state in this patient. Diaphragm contraction causes elevations in the rib cage and increases rib cage diameter, thus injuries to the phrenic nerves would again require other muscles of inspiration to adapt. The crural portion of the diaphragm would lose sensory innervation, however the costal portions would maintain sensory innervation as it is supplied by the adjacent intercostal nerves. The internal intercostal along with the abdominal muscles aid with active expiration and their function would not change.

Reference: pages 8–10

Answer 1.9.   **D**

Blood supply to the lungs is from the bronchial arteries and the pulmonary arteries. The bronchial arteries supply the walls of the bronchi and bronchioles to the level of the alveoli and arise from the aorta and intercostal arteries. Although important, the bronchial arteries only supply a minor portion of blood flow to the lungs while the pulmonary arteries supply the most. The communication of the deoxygenated pulmonary artery blood flow with the oxygenated bronchial artery blood flow, and their return to the heart, account for a normal shunt of as much as 5% of the cardiac output.

Reference: pages 15, 16

Answer 1.10.   **A-4, B-3, C-1, D-6, E-2, F-5**

Serous cells are secretory cells that secrete a variety of peptides including lysozyme, lactoferrin, and the secretory leukoprotease inhibitor. Mucus cells are other secretory cells that are important in chronic bronchitis. The ratio of the depth of gland penetration to the thickness of the bronchial wall (Reid index) is a measure of chronic bronchitis. Clara cells line the bronchioles and function as progenitors for ciliated cells, brush cells, and goblet cells. Kulchitsky cells are common in newborns and may be precursors of bronchial carcinoid tumors and small cell carcinomas. Pores of Kohn are holes that connect alveoli directly and Canals of Lambert are passages from the distal airways to adjacent alveoli. Both may play a role in preventing lung segments distal to obstructed airways from becoming atelectatic.

Reference: pages 14, 15

chapter 2

Pulmonary Circulation

QUESTIONS

Question 2.1. Which of the following is/are true regarding the pulmonary and bronchial vessels?

A. The main pulmonary artery wall is about one-third as thick as that of the aorta.
B. The cardiac output from the left ventricle is normally 1–2% higher than the cardiac output of the right ventricle as a result of the bronchial artery blood flow.
C. The bronchial arteries supply the visceral pleura while the pulmonary artery supplies the pericardium and tracheobronchial lymph nodes.
D. The vessels leaving the left heart are more compliant than the vessels leaving the right heart.
E. Structurally, the interstitial space that surrounds the pulmonary arteries and veins is continuous with the interstitial space around the capillaries in the alveolar septa.

Question 2.2. Which of the following statements is/are true concerning normal values obtained from a pulmonary artery catheter?

A. The mean pulmonary artery pressure is about 15 mm Hg with a further drop of 10 mm Hg across the alveolar capillary bed before entering the left atrium.
B. The pulmonary arterial end-diastolic pressure in normal subjects closely approximates the wedge pressure.
C. Pulmonary arterial pressure in normal subjects most closely approximates wedge pressure at the beginning of diastole.
D. At the end of diastole, the blood flow through the pulmonary circulation is less than at any other point in the cardiac cycle.

Question 2.3. Regarding the pulmonary blood volume and blood flow, which of the following statements is/are true?

A. With vigorous inhalation, up to one-fourth of a liter of blood can be expelled from the pulmonary circulation into the systemic circulation.
B. The blood flow through the lungs, in volume per unit time, can be calculated by dividing the oxygen consumption by the difference in the arterial and venous oxygen contents.
C. Using the thermal dilution technique, a cold indicator bolus is injected into the distal port of a pulmonary artery catheter to measure the cardiac output.
D. In the average human adult, the two lungs contain approximately 1 liter of blood.

Question 2.4. Which of the following statements is/are true regarding pulmonary blood flow and distribution?

A. Zone 1 has pulmonary alveolar pressures greater than pulmonary artery pressures.
B. Zone 3 has pulmonary alveolar pressures greater than pulmonary venous pressures.

C. In zone 2 the pulmonary venous pressures become greater than the alveolar pressures.

D. The perfusion gradient increases in zone 1 during exercise.

Question 2.5. **Pulmonary vascular resistance (PVR) has been described as the "input" pressure minus the "output" pressure divided by blood flow. Which of the following is/are true statements about the PVR when considering the pulmonary artery pressures and lung volumes?**

A. If pulmonary artery pressure is raised by increasing flow while lung volume and left atrial pressure are held constant, PVR increases.

B. If left atrial pressure is raised without allowing pulmonary artery pressure and blood flow to change, then PVR falls.

C. The caliber of capillaries is increased at higher lung volumes because of stretching of the alveolar walls.

D. With inflation to a high lung volume, alveolar pressure can rise with respect to perfusion pressure in capillaries.

Question 2.6. **Various mediators commonly found in the circulation have vasoconstrictive or vasodilatory effects. Regarding these substances, select the true statement(s) below.**

A. Alpha blockade with phentolamine will cause a slightly higher pulmonary vascular resistance.

B. Histamine causes vasoconstriction in the pulmonary vasculature.

C. Prostaglandins of the F series cause vasoconstriction, while those of the E series causes vasodilatation.

D. The most potent stimulus to pulmonary arterial vasoconstriction is hypercarbia.

E. Naturally occurring substances that are metabolically altered in the lungs include angiotensin II, bradykinin, and histamine.

Question 2.7. **Potent vasoactive factors are produced by the pulmonary vascular endothelial cells. Which of the following is/are correct regarding these factors and their regulation of pulmonary vascular tone?**

A. Nitric oxide is produced from L-arginine and produces vascular relaxation by increasing concentrations of cyclic guanosine 3',5'-monophosphate (cGMP).

B. Factors which stimulate the release of nitric oxide include acetylcholine, ATP, and bradykinin.

C. Angiotensin II is the most potent vasoconstricting agent known.

D. Endothelin-1 produces varying hemodynamic effects on different vascular beds but its most striking property is its sustained hypertensive action.

Question 2.8. **A 50-year-old man presents with respiratory distress. His pH is 7.30, $PaCO_2$ 30 mm Hg, and PaO_2 50 mm Hg on room air. Chest films reveal a right lower lobe consolidation with air bronchograms. Regarding hypoxic pulmonary vasoconstriction and its effects in this patient, which of the following is/are correct?**

A. In the systemic circulation, hypoxia produces vasodilatation, while in the pulmonary circulation, hypoxia results in vasoconstriction.

B. The vasoconstriction occurs on the arterial side of the pulmonary circulation when oxygen tension drops to approximately 60 mm Hg or less in the alveoli.

C. The vasoconstrictive response to a low alveolar PO_2 is reduced when the pH is reduced to 7.20.

D. Hypoxic pulmonary vasoconstriction increases blood flow to the poorly ventilated areas of the lung and thereby increases the degree of venous admixture and arterial hypoxemia.

Question 2.9. **Besides gas exchange, the lungs perform several metabolic functions. Which of the following is/are true when considering the metabolic demands of the lungs and the effects of various drugs after they pass through the lungs?**

A. Although diffusion in the lungs is an active process, it requires only minimal energy expenditure.
B. Essentially the entire metabolic cost of respiration is supplied by organs other than the lungs.
C. Substances that are almost completely removed or inactivated after a first pass through the lungs include angiotensin II and epinephrine.
D. Adenosine triphosphate and prostaglandin E_2 pass through the lungs without degradation or inactivation.

Question 2.10. **Various vasoactive substances are altered as they pass through the lungs. Match the vasoactive substances below with their respective descriptions.**

A. Serotonin
B. Histamine
C. Angiotensin
D. Bradykinin
E. Prostaglandins (E series)

1. Produced in mast cells and basophils, it is also a mediator of type I hypersensitivity.
2. Arachidonic acid derivative producing bronchial smooth muscle relaxation.
3. Felt to play a role in angioneurotic edema, this substance is about 80% inactivated in the lungs.
4. A decapeptide converted to its active form in the lungs.
5. A source of release is the argentaffin cells in the intestine; it is almost completely inactivated in the lungs.

ANSWERS

Answer 2.1. **A, B, E - True; C, D - False**

The pulmonary artery wall is thin, with a thickness approximately twice that of the vena cava and only one-third that of the aorta. It is also very distensible and compliant, averaging 3 ml/mm Hg, allowing the vessels leaving the right heart to be the most compliant. The bronchial arteries supply the lower part of the trachea, visceral pleura, pericardium, tracheobronchial lymph nodes, vasa vasorum of the pulmonary artery and vein, and the bronchi as far as the respiratory bronchioles. The blood leaving the bronchial arteries eventually enters the pulmonary veins and returns to the left atrium, causing a normal 1–2% increase in the left sided cardiac output over the right side. The interstitial space that surrounds the pulmonary arteries and veins is continuous with the interstitial space around the capillaries in the alveolar septa.

Reference: pages 25, 26

Answer 2.2.   **A, B, D - True; C - False**

The blood pressure within the pulmonary vasculature varies greatly depending upon the disease state. In normal subjects, the mean pulmonary artery pressure is about 15 mm Hg and is the highest pressure obtained throughout the pulmonary circulation. There is a successive drop down to about 5 mm Hg upon reaching the left atrium. The pulmonary artery end-diastolic pressure in normal subjects closely approximates the wedge pressure; however, any lung disease will change this relationship and diastolic pressures are therefore unreliable for use in wedge pressure approximations. The pulmonary artery diastolic pressure should be higher than the left atrial pressure allowing for a physiologic drop off across the pulmonary vascular bed. The pulmonary circulation is pulsatile, and flow is least at the end of diastole.

Reference: pages 26–28

Answer 2.3.   **B - True; A, C, D - False**

In the average adult, the two lungs contain approximately 450 ml of blood. Vigorous exhalation can expel over half of the blood from the lungs into the systemic circulation. The cardiac output, thus blood flow through the lung in volume per unit time, is defined in the Fick equation and is derived by dividing the oxygen consumption (VO_2) by the difference between the arterial oxygen content (CaO_2) and the mixed venous oxygen content (CvO_2). Cardiac output is also measured by the thermodilution technique. This technique uses a 10 ml bolus of cool liquid injected into the proximal part of a pulmonary artery catheter. A thermistor at the tip of the catheter senses a temperature change, which correlates with the volume of dilution by pulmonary blood flow.

Reference: pages 28–30

Answer 2.4.   **A - True; B, C, D - False**

Distribution of pulmonary blood flow is largely dependent on gravity. The lungs have been divided into three zones with the pressures as described: zone 1—pulmonary alveolar pressure > pulmonary artery pressure > pulmonary venous pressure; zone 2—pulmonary artery pressure > pulmonary alveolar pressure > pulmonary venous pressure; zone 3—pulmonary artery pressure > pulmonary venous pressure > pulmonary alveolar pressure. Zone 3 is the most "gravity dependent," and in the upright position, would be in the basilar segments of the lung, while in the supine position, zone three shifts to the posterior-dependent areas of the lungs. The zones are important when inserting a pulmonary artery catheter and then interpreting the data as the catheter tip may reflect alveolar pressures if placed in zone 1.

Reference: pages 29–31

Answer 2.5.   **B, D - True; A, C - False**

Pulmonary vascular resistance (PVR) is derived by subtracting the left atrial pressure from the mean pulmonary artery pressure and then dividing by the pulmonary blood flow in liters/min. Normally, PVR is only one-tenth the resistance of the systemic circulation. Normal pulmonary circulation has the ability to accommodate large increases in cardiac output with only a slight increase in pulmonary artery pressure. If pulmonary artery pressure is raised by increasing flow while lung volume and left atrial pressure are held constant, PVR decreases. Also, if left atrial pressure is raised without allowing pulmonary artery pressure and blood flow to change, then PVR falls. Vascular recruitment occurs at a critical opening pressure that must be exceeded in some arteries before they will conduct blood. The caliber of capillaries is reduced at higher lung volumes because of stretching of the alveolar walls.

Reference: pages 31–33

Answer 2.6. B, C, E - True; A, D - False

Regulation of the pulmonary vascular tone is maintained by various factors including the autonomic nervous system, catecholamines, and naturally occurring substances like histamine, angiotensin II, serotonin, and the prostaglandins. The alpha blockers will cause a decrease in pulmonary vascular resistance while histamine, by stimulating the H_1 receptors, causes vasoconstriction. Prostaglandins of the F series will cause vasoconstriction while the E series has the opposite effect. Of all the mediators, the most potent stimulus for pulmonary artery vasoconstriction is hypoxia. There is a complex interrelationship among all of the various mediators with only a few listed above. A wide variety of vasoactive mediators are produced and metabolized in the lungs.

Reference: pages 33, 34

Answer 2.7. A, B, D - True; C - False

Various substances are produced in the vascular endothelial cells which regulate pulmonary vascular tone. Two substances that are currently the center of much research are nitric oxide and endothelin-1. Nitric oxide is produced by nitric oxide synthase from L-arginine, producing vascular relaxation by increasing cGMP. Nitric oxide is released by factors that bind to receptors on the endothelial cell wall (including acetylcholine, ATP, and bradykinin). In opposition to nitric oxide, endothelin-1 produces vasoconstriction and is the most potent vasoconstricting agent yet discovered (10 times the potency of angiotensin II). Its role in the regulation of normal pulmonary vascular tone is still unclear.

Reference: pages 34, 35

Answer 2.8. A, B - True; C, D - False

Hypoxemia is the most potent pulmonary arterial vasoconstrictor; however, in the systemic circulation, it produces vasodilatation. Vasoconstriction within the pulmonary arteries due to hypoxia occurs prealveolar (arterial side) when the PAO_2 is approximately 60 mm Hg or less. Acidosis potentates hypoxic pulmonary vasoconstriction. A PAO_2 of 40 mm Hg has been shown to double the effects of vasoconstriction in the pulmonary artery when the pH is lowered to 7.20 in some animals. Hypoxic pulmonary vasoconstriction is a useful adaptation, decreasing blood flow to the poorly ventilated areas of the lung and thereby reducing the degree of venous admixture and arterial hypoxemia.

Reference: pages 36, 37

Answer 2.9. B - True; A, C, D - False

Most of the work required for gas exchange is provided by the respiratory muscles and the heart, thus essentially the entire metabolic cost of respiration is supplied by organs other than the lungs. Diffusion is a passive process requiring no energy; however, it is estimated that 4–5% of resting whole-body oxygen consumption is consumed by the lungs. Many substances are inactivated by passing through the lungs, including prostaglandin E_2 and adenosine triphosphate; others, such as angiotensin II and epinephrine, are unaffected. A more complete listing is found in Table 2.2, *Chest Medicine,* 3rd edition.

Reference: page 37

Answer 2.10.   **A - 5, B - 1, C - 4, D - 3, E - 2**

Several of the vasoactive substances that play a role in regulating pulmonary vascular tone are degraded while passing through the lungs. Serotonin is broken down before leaving the lungs. It is derived from the argentaffin cells in the intestine as well as from platelets. Histamine, produced in tissue mast cells and basophils, remains unaffected after entry into the lungs. Angiotensin I is converted to its active form angiotensin II by the pulmonary circulation. Bradykinin is about 80% inactivated. It is felt to play a role in bronchial asthma and anaphylaxis. The arachidonic acid metabolites (prostaglandins, prostacyclin, and thromboxane A_2) have mixed functions. The F series prostaglandins initiate pulmonary artery vasoconstriction while the E series produce vasodilatation.

Reference: pages 37–39

chapter 3

Mechanics of Respiration

QUESTIONS

Question 3.1. **Which of the following statements is/are correct regarding total lung capacity (TLC)?**

A. Total lung capacity will be increased if the chest wall becomes more compliant.
B. Total lung capacity is the volume at which maximal negative pressure generated by inspiratory muscles is equal to the relaxed positive pressure of the respiratory system.
C. Total lung capacity is the total amount of air that is in the lung after maximal inspiration.
D. Total lung capacity is dependent on the height, age, and sex of the subject.

Question 3.2. **Which of the following statements is/are correct regarding pleural pressures?**

A. Pleural pressure is the pressure at the inner surface of the chest wall and the outer surface of the lung.
B. The main factors responsible for the pleural pressure gradient are gravity, mismatching of the shapes of the chest wall and lung, and the weight of intrathoracic structures.
C. Pleural pressure can be estimated via esophageal balloon pressure measurements.
D. Pleural pressures are constant throughout the lung.

Question 3.3. **Which of the following statements is/are correct regarding the role of surfactant in the normal lung?**

A. Surfactant is secreted by type II pneumocytes present in the alveoli.
B. Surfactant helps promote alveolar stability.
C. Surfactant decreases the surface tension of alveoli, thereby reducing the transpulmonary pressure necessary to achieve a given lung volume.
D. The presence of surfactant assists in the lung response to infection.

Question 3.4. **When considering the patterns of air flow present in the lung, which of the following statements is/are correct?**

A. Laminar air flow is dependent on the density of a gas.
B. Transitional air flow is dependent on both density and viscosity of a gas.
C. Turbulent air flow is dependent on the viscosity of a gas.
D. Laminar air flow occurs in small airways, whereas turbulent flow occurs mainly in the trachea.

Question 3.5. **Which of the following conditions result(s) in a decrease in the distensibility properties of the lung:**

A. Interstitial fibrosis
B. Pulmonary hypertension

C. Adult respiratory distress syndrome (ARDS)
D. Emphysema

Question 3.6. **Which of the following statements is/are correct regarding the origin of elastic recoil in the normal excised lung?**

A. During inflation, most of the pressure of elastic recoil is due to surface tension.
B. During inflation, a linear relationship exists between the pressure needed for distension and the percent of total lung capacity achieved.
C. During deflation, most of the pressure of elastic recoil results from the elastic properties of the lung itself.
D. Surface tension is a true force which affects elastic recoil.

Question 3.7. **Which of the following statements is/are correct concerning the use of helium-oxygen mixture (He-O$_2$) in the evaluation of air flow in the lungs?**

A. The use of He-O$_2$ flow-volume loops is most useful in detecting disease of small peripheral airways.
B. He-O$_2$ has become a useful tool because it is easy to use and there is little variability among both subjects and interpretation of the findings.
C. The use of He-O$_2$ during FEV maneuvers allows detection of abnormalities in smokers when their Vmax is still within normal range.
D. A mixture of 80% helium and 20% oxygen has a viscosity approximately one-third that of air, making it useful in evaluating laminar flow.

Question 3.8. **Distribution of ventilation depends on which of the following factor(s)?**

A. Tissue interdependence
B. Collateral ventilation
C. Regional differences in pleural pressures
D. Time constants of the respiratory units

Question 3.9. **Which of the following statements are TRUE/FALSE regarding airway resistance in the lung?**

A. The major portion of airway resistance resides in narrow peripheral airways.
B. During nasal breathing, less than one-third of the total resistance is offered by the nasal passages.
C. Nasal resistance increases disproportionately with increasing flow rates.
D. Airway resistance depends on the number, length, and cross-sectional area of airways, with cross-sectional area being the most important determinant.

Question 3.10. **(TRUE/FALSE) Airway resistance is increased by the following conditions:**

A. Parasympathetic stimulation of bronchial smooth muscle
B. Sympathetic stimulation of bronchial smooth muscle
C. Stimulation of irritant receptors
D. Mucosal edema
E. Mucous gland hyperplasia

Question 3.11. **The following conditions will lead to an increase in residual volume (TRUE/FALSE):**

A. Strengthening of respiratory muscles.
B. Decreased compliance of the chest wall.
C. Decreased compliance of the lung.

Question 3.12. **The following statements are TRUE/FALSE regarding mechanical work necessary for adequate alveolar ventilation:**

A. Individuals with pulmonary fibrosis tend to breathe more deeply and slowly.
B. Individuals with emphysema usually have rapid and shallow breathing.
C. Oxygen cost of breathing can be measured by determining total O_2 consumption of the body at rest and during hyperventilation.
D. The oxygen cost of breathing accounts for 3–5% of total O_2 consumption.
E. Large tidal volumes increase elastic work of breathing, whereas rapid breathing increases work against flow-restrictive forces.

Question 3.13. **Which one of the following statements is incorrect regarding subdivisions of lung volumes?**

A. Total lung capacity equals vital capacity plus residual volume.
B. Total lung capacity equals inspiratory capacity plus functional residual capacity.
C. Total lung capacity equals inspiratory reserve volume plus functional residual capacity.
D. Total lung capacity equals inspiratory capacity plus expiratory reserve volume plus residual volume.

Question 3.14. **The maximum flow rate (Vmax) on expiration is NOT dependent on which one of the following?**

A. Elastic recoil of the lung
B. Tendency of the airways to collapse
C. Resistance of the upstream segment
D. Resistance of the downstream segment

Question 3.15. **Match the lung disease with the predominant mechanism leading to reduced flow rates:**

1. Emphysema
2. Asthma
3. Chronic bronchitis

A. Tendency of airways to collapse
B. Decreased elastic recoil
C. Increased resistance of upstream segments

ANSWERS

Answer 3.1. **All are correct**

Total lung capacity is defined as the total amount of air that is in the lungs after maximal inspiration. TLC is also the volume at which the maximal negative pressure generated by the inspiratory muscles is equal to the relaxed positive pressure of the respiratory system (see Figure 3.4, page 45 in Chest Medicine, 3rd edition). Accordingly, the total lung capacity will be reduced if the lung or the chest wall become stiffer (less compliant) or if the inspiratory muscles become weaker. Conversely, the TLC will be increased if the lungs or chest wall become more compliant or if the muscles become stronger. The TLC is dependent on the height, age, and sex of the subject, being larger in taller, younger, and male individuals.

Reference: pages 43–45

Answer 3.2.   **A, B, C**

Pleural pressure is defined as the pressure at the inner surface of the chest wall and the outer surface of the lungs. Direct measurement of the pleural pressure is not usually done due to the danger of producing a pneumothorax or an infection of the pleural space. At the present time, pleural pressures are usually measured indirectly using a balloon placed in the patient's esophagus. Since the esophagus is located between the two pleural spaces, esophageal pressure measurements provide a close approximation of the pleural pressure at the level of the balloon in the thorax. Although estimation of the pleural pressure via an esophageal balloon gives a value for the pleural pressure, the pleural pressure is not uniform throughout the chest. There is a gradient in pleural pressure between the top and bottom of the lung, with the pleural pressure being lowest or most negative at the top and highest or least negative at the bottom. The main factors responsible for this gradient are probably gravity, mismatching of the shapes of the chest wall and lung, and the weight of the lungs and other intrathoracic structures.

Reference: page 46

Answer 3.3.   **All are correct**

Surfactant is a complex mixture composed of lipids, proteins, and carbohydrates, secreted by the type II pneumocytes that are present in the alveoli. When surfactant is present, surface tension decreases dramatically as the surface area is decreased, thereby promoting alveolar stability and reducing the transpulmonary pressure necessary to achieve a given lung volume. The presence of surfactant also increases the antibacterial capabilities of alveolar macrophages and modulates lymphocyte responsiveness.

Reference: pages 48–49

Answer 3.4.   **B, D**

Air flow through a tube can be either laminar or turbulent. Laminar flow is organized, and streamlines are everywhere parallel to the sides of the tube. Laminar flow is dependent on the viscosity of a gas but is independent of its density. Turbulent flow occurs at high rates and is characterized by a complete disorganization of the streamlines so that molecules of gas move laterally, collide with one another, and change their velocities. With turbulent flow the viscosity of the gas becomes unimportant, but an increase in gas density increases the pressure drop for a given flow. In the lung, laminar flow occurs only in the small peripheral airways, where, owing to the large overall cross-sectional area, flow through any given airway is extremely slow. Turbulent flow occurs in the trachea. In the remainder of the lung, flow is neither laminar nor turbulent, but rather mixed or transitional. With a transitional flow pattern, flow is dependent on both the viscosity and the density of the gas.

Reference: pages 50–51

Answer 3.5.   **A, B, C**

The lungs of patients with interstitial fibrosis are less distensible than normal lungs because the tissue retractive forces are increased. The stiffness of the lung may also be increased when the pulmonary vessels are engorged with blood (pulmonary hypertension) or when the interstitial spaces are filled with fluid (ARDS). The lungs of patients with emphysema are actually more distensible because many alveolar walls have been destroyed, resulting in a loss of elastic elements.

Reference: page 48

Answer 3.6. **A, C**

The total force causing the inflated lung to recoil inward has two components: the first arises from the elastic properties of the lung itself and the second arises from surface tension. On inflation, much more elastic recoil is due to surface tension than is due to elastic properties of the lung. Alternatively, during deflation the majority of elastic recoil is due to the lungs' inherent elasticity. When the normal lung is deflated and then inflated with air, the volume increases very little until a pressure of about 8 cm H_2O is reached. At pressures above this, the volume increases rapidly until the TLC is approached at about 30 cm H_2O. The filling of the lung is uneven, as some areas of the lung are seen to inflate rapidly. Surface tension does not represent a true force, but arises because any surface has a tendency to decrease to a minimum.

Reference: pages 48–50

Answer 3.7. **A, C**

In the normal lung during forced expiration, flow in the peripheral airways is laminar, flow in the medium-sized airways is transitional, and flow in the large airways is turbulent. Only laminar flow is independent of gas density. In normal subjects, flow at low volumes is density independent because the collapsible segments of the lung are more peripheral and the flow rates lower. A mixture of 80% helium and 20% oxygen has a viscosity that is very similar to that of air, but a density that is approximately one-third of air. The use of He-O_2 flow-volume loops has its greatest utility in detecting disease of the small peripheral airways. Since the small airways usually contribute a minor portion of the total airway resistance, changes in these airways may not be detectable by measurements of airway resistance. Studies in both smokers and non-smokers using flow-volume loops with air and He-O_2 have shown that the use of He-O_2 during an FEV maneuver allows the detection of functional abnormalities in smokers at a stage when their Vmax is still within the normal range while they are breathing room air. The utilization of He-O_2 flow-volume loops in clinical pulmonary disease has proven difficult in healthy subjects and patients because of large intrasubject and intersubject variability and variability in interpretation of the same series of curves by different observers.

Reference: pages 57, 58

Answer 3.8. **All are correct**

The lung has a connective tissue framework containing elastic elements. Because contiguous units are attached to each other, they are not free to move independently. This dependence of one respiratory unit on the movements of its neighbors is called tissue interdependence. Collateral ventilation is ventilation of the alveolar structures through passages that bypass the normal airways. Without collateral ventilation, alveoli distal to obstructed airways would become atelectatic. The possible pathways for collateral ventilation include intraalveolar communications (pores of Kohn), bronchiole-alveolar communications (canals of Lambert), and the interbronchiolar communications of Martin. Collateral ventilation may be very important in preserving the uniformity of ventilation in patients with emphysema and other lung diseases. The time constant of a respiratory unit is the time it takes to reach 37% of its original volume, based exponentially on both the resistance and compliance of the respiratory system. In patients with peripheral airways disease, the time constants of some respiratory units are increased, so that with more rapid breathing, equilibration between alveolar and mouth pressure does not occur at either end-inspiration or end-expiration, leading to alterations in distribution of ventilation. The variation seen in pleural pressures results from gravity, mismatching shapes of the lung and chest wall, and weight of intrathoracic structures. Since alveolar pressure is constant throughout the lungs, the effect of the pleural pressure gradient is that different parts of the lung have different distending pressures. At low lung volumes, the pleural pressure may become positive in the lower regions of the lung, compressing airways and resulting in alveoli that are not ventilated.

Reference: pages 46–47, 58–59

Answer 3.9.   **C, D - True; A, B - False**

During nasal breathing, the resistance offered by the nose is the largest single component, constituting one-half to two-thirds of the total resistance at low flow rates. The nasal resistance increases disproportionately with increasing flow rates, so during heavy exercise one switches from nasal breathing to mouth breathing. Airway resistance depends on the number, length, and cross-sectional area of the conducting airways. Since resistance to flow in a given airway changes according to the 4th power of the radius, the cross-sectional area within the tracheobronchial tree is by far the most important determinant of airway resistance. This explains why resistance does not increase disproportionately in the periphery of the tracheobronchial tree where airways become successively narrower, as the branching results in an increased average cross-sectional diameter of peripheral airways.

Reference: pages 51–52

Answer 3.10.   **A, C, D, E - True; B - False**

Contraction of bronchial smooth muscle narrows the airways and increases airway resistance. The tone of bronchial smooth muscle is under the control of the autonomic nervous system. Sympathetic stimulation causes bronchodilation (decreasing resistance), while parasympathetic stimulation causes bronchoconstriction (increasing resistance). Stimulation of irritant receptors in the tracheobronchial tree induces bronchoconstriction reflexly via the parasympathetic nerve fibers contained in the vagus nerve (increasing resistance). In patients with lung disease, mucosal edema, hypertrophy and hyperplasia of mucous glands, increased production of mucus, and hypertrophy of the bronchial smooth muscle all tend to decrease airway caliber and contribute to the increased airway resistance.

Reference: Page 52

Answer 3.11.   **B - True; A, C - False**

The residual volume (RV) is the volume at which the maximal positive airway pressure is equal to the relaxed negative pressure of the respiratory system. The RV will increase if there is expiratory muscle weakness, or if the pressure-volume curve of the respiratory system is shifted to the left, which can occur with a noncompliant chest wall or a very compliant lung.

Reference: page 45

Answer 3.12.   **C, D, E - True; A, B - False**

The work of breathing at any given level of alveolar ventilation is dependent on the pattern of breathing. Several studies have shown that both normal individuals and patients with lung disease adopt the respiratory pattern at which work is minimal. Individuals with pulmonary fibrosis, which is characterized by increased elastic work of breathing, tend to breathe rapidly and shallowly. Individuals with airway obstruction, which is characterized by increased nonelastic work of breathing, usually breathe more slowly and deeply. The oxygen cost of breathing can be measured by determining the total oxygen consumption of the body at rest and at increased levels of ventilation produced by voluntary hyperventilation. In normal subjects the oxygen cost of breathing is on the order of 0.5–1.0 ml per liter of ventilation and therefore accounts for 3–5% of the total oxygen consumption.

Reference: pages 60–61

Answer 3.13 C

Total lung capacity is defined as the total amount of air in the lungs after maximal inspiration. This amount can be subdivided based on the vital capacity, which is the maximal amount of air that a subject is able to expire after maximal inspiration, plus the residual volume, which is the amount of air that is still in the lungs at the end of maximal expiration (answer A). It can also be divided into the inspiratory capacity, which is the maximal volume of air that can be inspired from the resting level plus the functional residual capacity, which is the quantity of air in the lungs and airways at the end of a spontaneous expiration, or resting level (answer B). The functional residual capacity can be subdivided into the expiratory reserve volume, which is the maximum amount of air that can be expired beyond the functional residual capacity plus the residual volume (answer D). Answer C is incorrect because it adds the inspiratory reserve volume, which is the maximal amount of air that can be inspired beyond the tidal volume, plus the functional residual capacity, or the amount after expiration, thus omitting the amount of gas contained in the tidal volume.

Reference: pages 43–44

Answer 3.14: D

Vmax can be obtained through the following formula based on the work of Pride et al., where

$$\text{Vmax} = \frac{\text{Pst(L)} \times \text{Ptm}'}{\text{Rs}}$$

When analyzed, it is seen that Vmax depends on three different factors: (*a*) the elastic recoil of the lung (Pst(L)), (*b*) the tendency of the airways to collapse (Ptm'), and (*c*) the resistance of the upstream segments (Rs).

Reference: page 56

Answer 3.15. 1-B; 2-A; 3-C

Emphysema, asthma, and chronic bronchitis are the three main diseases that cause reduced flow rates on expiration. With emphysema, the main abnormality is decreased elastic recoil of the lungs; with chronic bronchitis, the predominant abnormality is increased resistance of the upstream segment; while with asthma, the constriction of the bronchial smooth muscles greatly increases the tendency of the airways to collapse, and thereby reduces flow rates by this mechanism. Of course with all three diseases, all the factors interact to some extent to produce reduced expiratory flow rates.

Reference: page 56

chapter 4

Ventilation, Gas Transfer, and Oxygen Delivery

QUESTIONS

Question 4.1. **Which of the following statements is/are correct regarding normal anatomic shunting of blood through the pulmonary circulation?**

A. One to three percent of mixed venous blood flows into the systemic circulation without perfusing the alveoli.
B. Normal anatomic shunting may occur through the bronchial, mediastinal, and the left thebesian veins.
C. In older subjects (>60 years of age) the PAO_2-PaO_2 difference increases as changes occur in ventilation and perfusion.
D. In normal subjects aged 21–30, the average PAO_2–PaO_2 difference is 5–10 mm Hg.

Question 4.2. **Which of the following statements is/are correct regarding arterial hypoxemia?**

A. A defect in gas transfer due to diffusion limitation does not occur in normal humans.
B. In patients who are hypoxemic and retaining CO_2, inadequate alveolar ventilation alone can explain an elevated alveolar to arterial oxygen difference.
C. Ventilation/perfusion mismatch is the most common cause of hypoxemia in patients with lung disease.
D. Acute lung injuries, such as ARDS, cause severe hypoxemia predominantly due to ventilation/perfusion mismatching.

Question 4.3. **Which of the following statements is/are correct regarding physiologic responses to increased oxygen demand?**

A. When mixed venous O_2 drops below 30 mm Hg, cells switch from aerobic to anaerobic metabolism.
B. Lactic acid production improves O_2 uptake by tissues.
C. An early mechanism to compensate for a decrease in cardiac output is an increase in 2,3-DPG.
D. Responses to acute increases in oxygen demand are more efficient in improving O_2 delivery than are responses to chronically increased oxygen demand.

Question 4.4. **Which of the following condition(s) shift the carbon dioxide (CO_2) dissociation curve to the right in a normal subject with a normal percent saturated hemoglobin?**

A. Polycythemia
B. Anemia

C. Oxygenation
D. Hypoxemia

Question 4.5. **Which of the following is the most common cause of hypoxemia in patients with lung disease?**

A. Hypoventilation
B. Diffusion defects
C. Ventilation-perfusion mismatch
D. Right to left shunts

Question 4.6. **A normal subject breathing room air at sea level has the following arterial blood values: pH 7.41, PaO2 90, PaCO2 40. Calculate the alveolar PO2 (PAO2) and alveolar-arterial oxygen difference:**

A. $PAO_2 = 100$ mm Hg; $PAO_2 - PaO2 = 60$ mm Hg
B. $PAO_2 = 150$ mm Hg; $PAO_2 - PaO_2 = 20$ mm Hg
C. $PAO_2 = 150$ mm Hg; $PAO_2 - PaO_2 = 60$ mm Hg
D. $PAO_2 = 150$ mm Hg; $PAO_2 - PaO_2 = 10$ mm Hg
E. $PAO_2 = 100$ mm Hg; $PAO_2 - PaO_2 = 10$ mm Hg

Question 4.7. **Positive end-expiratory pressure (PEEP) improves arterial oxygenation by all of the following means EXCEPT:**

A. Redistribution of lung water
B. Reduction of flow to shunt vessels
C. Extending expiratory time
D. Recruitment of atelectatic lung tissue

Question 4.8. **A patient has the following hemodynamic and respiratory findings: cardiac index of 3.2, cardiac output of 5.0 liters/min, hemoglobin 13.6 g/dl, and a calculated hemoglobin saturation of 96%. His arterial pH is 7.41, PaO_2 79, and $PaCO_2$ 41. Calculate this patient's systemic oxygen transport.**

A. 417 ml/min
B. 547 ml/min
C. 652 ml/min
D. 719 ml/min
E. 875 ml/min

Question 4.9. **Which of the following statements are TRUE/FALSE regarding ventilation/perfusion relationships?**

A. There is normally a gradient of both ventilation and perfusion from the top to the bottom of the lung.
B. The effects of true shunts can be estimated by measuring the PaO_2 while the patient breathes 100% oxygen.
C. There is a decreasing ratio of ventilation to perfusion on descending from the apex to the base of the lungs.
D. Arterial PO_2 primarily reflects areas of the lung with relatively low ventilation/perfusion ratios.

Question 4.10. **Which of the following statements are TRUE/FALSE concerning diffusion of gases in the lung?**

A. The difference in gas tensions is the driving force for diffusion.
B. During exercise, the diffusion capacity for oxygen may increase to three times the normal level at rest.

C. The DLCO must fall to about 10% of the predicted value before changes occur in PaO_2 at rest.

D. Abnormal diffusion plays a large role in hypoxia seen in patients with lung disease.

Question 4.11. **TRUE/FALSE - The following conditions cause a shift of the oxyhemoglobin dissociation curve to the right (increasing oxygen delivery at tissue level):**

A. Increased levels of 2,3-DPG
B. Increased temperature
C. Increased pH
D. Increased levels of carbon monoxide

Question 4.12. **Which of the following statements are TRUE/FALSE regarding the role of the erythropoietic system in oxygen delivery?**

A. Increasing the hemoglobin levels above normal will always result in improved oxygen delivery.
B. The most common abnormality of the erythropoietic system is abnormal hemoglobin production.
C. In cases of carbon monoxide poisoning, patients die due to tissue hypoxia.
D. The principal response to chronic anemia is increased heart rate and pulse pressures.
E. Chronic anemia results in a decrease of red cell 2,3-DPG

Question 4.13. **Determine whether the oxyhemoglobin dissociation curve would be shifted *(A)* to the left, *(B)* to the right, or *(C)* unchanged, by the following conditions.**

1. 34-year-old woman with acute carbon monoxide poisoning.
2. 18-year-old man with hypothermia after prolonged exposure.
3. 56-year-old man with acute anterior myocardial infarction with a cardiac output of 3.0 liters/min.
4. 22-year-old woman who has homozygous SS disease (sickle trait).
5. 45-year-old woman with diabetic ketoacidosis.

ANSWERS

Answer 4.1. **All are correct**

There is a difference in alveolar and arterial PO_2 as a result of normal anatomic shunting, through which 1–3% of mixed venous blood flows directly into the systemic circulation without perfusing the alveolar capillaries. This occurs mainly through the bronchial, mediastinal, and left thebesian veins. In normal subjects 21–30 years of age, the average alveolar-arterial difference is 5–10 mm Hg. With the normal aging process, there are gradually more and more lung units with uneven ventilation and perfusion. Thus, in normal adults 61–75 years of age, the average alveolar-arterial oxygen difference increases, and may go as high as 30 mm Hg in normal subjects.

Reference: page 64

Answer 4.2. **A, C**

A defect in gas transfer due to diffusion limitation does not occur in normal humans at sea level because even at high cardiac outputs the blood remains in the capillaries long enough for adequate equilibrium. In patients who are hypoxemic and retaining CO_2, the relative contribution to the hypoxemia of alveolar hypoventilation can be determined by calculating alveolar-arterial PO_2 difference. If this is normal, one can assume that the observed hypoxemia can be corrected by achieving adequate alveolar ventilation. If, however, the PAO_2-PaO_2 difference is elevated, then there is a defect in gas transfer (usually a V/Q mismatch) in addition to the hypoventilation. Ventilation-perfusion mismatch is the most common cause of hypoxemia in patients with lung disease. Acute lung injuries cause severe hypoxemia mostly as a result of increased right to left shunting.

Reference: pages 72–73

Answer 4.3.   **A, B, C**

If oxygen delivery is reduced because of a decrease in cardiac output, hemoglobin concentration, or gas exchange, the tissues respond by extracting additional oxygen from the capillary blood. When the mixed venous O_2 (PVO_2) drops below about 30 mm Hg, the cells switch from aerobic to anaerobic metabolism to supply their energy needs. Oxygen delivery is markedly affected by a reduction in cardiac output. The immediate compensatory mechanism for a low cardiac output is increased extraction of oxygen from blood that perfuses the tissues, facilitated by an increase in red blood cell 2,3-DPG, which displaces oxygen on the hemoglobin molecule and allows more oxygen to be extracted. If this fails to meet tissue demands, anaerobic metabolism occurs and lactate is produced, causing a drop in pH and a further shift to the right of the oxyhemoglobin dissociation curve. In general, responses to chronic increases in oxygen demand are more efficient, since the body has more time to adjust.

Reference: pages 74–75

Answer 4.4.   **A, C**

While arterial PO_2 is dependent on several factors that affect gas exchange, arterial PCO_2 is dependent solely on the relationship of CO_2 production to alveolar ventilation. In normal subjects, the CO_2 dissociation curve is relatively flat in the physiologic range. The curve shifts to the right with polycythemia and to the left with anemia, due to the presence or absence of hemoglobin binding sites. Oxygenation shifts the curve to the right as CO_2 is displaced from the hemoglobin sites by oxygen, whereas hypoxia shifts the curve to the left.

Reference: pages 65–66

Answer 4.5.   **C**

Hypoventilation causes hypoxemia due to its effects on the alveolar PO_2. Usually, this hypoxemia can be corrected by achieving adequate alveolar ventilation. Three factors decrease oxygen diffusion and cause hypoxemia: a decrease in the lung diffusion capacity for oxygen; a decrease in the oxygen gradient between alveoli and capillary blood; and a decrease in equilibrium time. Two or more of these abnormalities must be present for diffusion defects to become a factor in hypoxemia. Diffusion defects are easily corrected by increasing the inspired FIO_2. True right to left shunts may also cause hypoxemia, but these are more commonly seen in acute lung injuries with severe lung damage. Ventilation-perfusion mismatching is the most common cause of hypoxemia in patients with lung disease.

Reference: pages 70–72

Answer 4.6.   **E**

PAO_2 can be calculated using the following formula:
$$PAO_2 = PIO_2 - \frac{PaCO_2}{R}$$
where PIO_2 is the partial pressure of inspired oxygen, $PaCO_2$ is the arterial PCO_2 (which is substituted for the alveolar PCO_2 since they are assumed to be identical), and R is the respiratory exchange ratio (estimated as 0.8). With the patient breathing room air (21% oxygen) at sea level (barometric pressure 760 mm Hg and normal body temperature of 37°C), water vapor is 47 mm Hg. The equation then becomes:
$$PAO_2 = 0.21\ (760 - 47) - 40/0.8$$
$$= 0.21\ (713) - 50$$
$$= 150 - 50$$
$$= 100 \text{ mm Hg}$$
The difference between alveolar and arterial oxygen tensions can then be calculated by subtracting the measured PaO_2 (90 mm Hg) from the calculated PAO_2 (100 mm Hg) to give an alveolar-arterial oxygen difference of 10 mm Hg.

Reference: pages 66–67

Answer 4.7.   **C**

Positive end-expiratory pressure increases end-expiratory lung volumes and tends to improve arterial oxygenation by at least three mechanisms: recruitment of atelectatic lung tissue, redistribution of lung water, and reduction of flow to shunt vessels. Similar mechanisms are likely to operate in all techniques that elevate mean airway pressure. PEEP does not have any effect on expiratory time.

Reference: page 73

Answer 4.8.   **E**

Systemic oxygen transport, or the amount of oxygen delivered to the tissues and metabolized per minute, can be calculated by multiplying the cardiac output (Q) by the arterial blood oxygen content (CaO_2):
$$\text{Systemic } O_2 \text{ transport (ml/min)} = Q \text{ (liter/min)} \times CaO_2 \text{ (ml/liter)}$$
$$= Q \times (\text{grams hemoglobin} \times 1.34 \text{ ml } O_2/g) \times SaO_2$$
$$= 5000 \text{ ml/min} \times (0.136 \text{ g/ml x } 1.34 \text{ ml } O_2/g \times 0.96)$$
$$= 875 \text{ ml/min}$$

Reference: page 73

Answer 4.9.   **A, B, C, D, - True**

In the upright position, blood flow increases progressively from the top to the bottom of the lungs. Because of the movement of the diaphragm and larger pressure changes with inspiration around the lower lobe, ventilation also increases from top to bottom, but not as much as perfusion. Thus, there is normally a gradient of both ventilation and perfusion from the top to the bottom of the lungs. Since blood flow increases relatively more from apex to lung base than does ventilation, there is a decreasing ratio of ventilation to perfusion on descending from the apex to the base of the lung. The gas exchange units near the lung bases, where perfusion is relatively high and ventilation/perfusion ratios relatively low, contribute much more to the arterial blood, and since their effects predominate, arterial PO_2 primarily reflects areas with relatively low ventilation/perfusion relationships. The portion of venous admixture caused by true right to left shunts can be separated from that due to poorly ventilated lung units by having the subject breathe 100% oxygen for at least 15 minutes and then calculating the resultant change in shunt fraction.

Reference: pages 68–69

Answer 4.10. **A, B, C - True; D - False**

Gas transfer across the alveolar-capillary membrane occurs by passive diffusion, which is related to the partial pressures of these gases in the alveoli and in the pulmonary capillaries. The difference in oxygen and CO_2 tensions across the membrane represents the driving pressure for diffusion for each gas. During exercise, diffusion capacity for oxygen may increase by more than three times through pulmonary capillary recruitment and an increase in capillary blood volume. The diffusion capacity must fall to about 10% of the predicted value before any change in arterial oxygen at rest will occur. For practical purposes, abnormal diffusion plays only a minor role in the hypoxemia seen in patients with lung diseases. This role is of even less importance, since it can be corrected by small increases in the inspired oxygen.

Reference: page 70

Answer 4.11. **A, B, D - True; C - False**

A decrease in blood pH is associated with a shift in the curve to the right; thus, at higher pH levels found in the lungs, oxygen is bound more easily, while at lower pH levels found in tissues, oxygen is freed more easily. Lower temperatures shift the curve to the left, while higher temperatures shift the curve to the right. The binding capacity for oxygen is also affected by an increase or decrease in the 2,3-diphosphoglycerate content of the red cells. Since the 2,3-DPG competes with oxygen for sites on the hemoglobin molecule, increased levels of 2,3-DPG shift the curve to the right and allow for improved oxygen delivery. Carbon monoxide binds extremely readily with hemoglobin to form carboxyhemoglobin. This decreases the ability of the hemoglobin to carry oxygen, shifting the curve to the right.

Reference: pages 74–75

Answer 4.12. **C, D - True; A, B, E - False**

The normal hematocrit of 40–50% is optimum for maximum O_2 delivery. An increase in the hematocrit will increase the oxygen carrying capacity of blood within certain limits; however, as the hematocrit rises above 55%, cardiac output falls and the polycythemia becomes a self-defeating mechanism. The most common abnormality of the erythropoietic system is blood loss, either acute or chronic. Carbon monoxide poisoning causes acute failure of the erythropoietic system by decreasing oxygen saturation. Victims die of tissue hypoxia because the hemoglobin is not available for oxygen transport. The principal response to a chronic decrease in circulating red cells (anemia) is an increased heart rate and pulse pressure with a resultant rise in cardiac output. With chronic anemia, there is also an increase in red cell 2,3-DPG with an accompanying shift of the oxyhemoglobin curve to the right, which decreases hemoglobin-oxygen affinity and makes oxygen more available to the tissues.

Reference: page 77

Answer 4.13.   **1-B; 2-A; 3-B; 4-C; 5-B**

Due to its high affinity for binding to the hemoglobin molecule, carbon monoxide shifts the oxyhemoglobin curve to the right. Decreased body temperature will shift the curve to the left. Decreased cardiac output will lead to an increase in red blood cell 2,3-DPG, shifting the curve to the right. Presence of sickle cell trait, in and of itself, has no effect on the dissociation curve. A decrease in pH as seen with diabetic ketoacidosis will cause a shift to the right.

Reference: pages 74–75

Diagnostic Studies in Patients with Respiratory Problems

chapter 5

History and Physical Examination

QUESTIONS

Question 5.1. **Which of the following statements is/are correct regarding extrapulmonary signs of lung disease:**

A. Hypoxemia is associated with cyanosis if 5 g/dl or more of reduced hemoglobin is present.
B. Central cyanosis implies involvement of gas transfer in the lungs.
C. Peripheral cyanosis without central cyanosis implies a circulatory problem.
D. Clubbing is always associated with lung disease.

Question 5.2. **Which of the following statements is/are correct regarding pleural friction rubs?**

A. Pleural rubs are generally loud, and sound as though they are just below the site of auscultation.
B. Pleural rubs often occur simultaneously with complaint of chest pain.
C. Pleural rubs are a series of small explosions, rather than a single coarse sound.
D. Pleural rubs occur exclusively during inspiration.

Question 5.3. **Which of the following statements is/are correct regarding the observance of hemoptysis?**

A. It is important to quantitate hemoptysis, as well as observing for color and presence of clots.
B. The most frequently observed cause of hemoptysis is chronic bronchitis.
C. Hemoptysis can be differentiated from hematemesis based on pH, presence of blood streaking, and presence of food particles.
D. In up to one-third of the cases, the cause of hemoptysis is unknown.

Question 5.4. **Which of the following statements is/are correct regarding sputum induction and gastric lavage?**

A. If patients are unable to produce sputum, inhalation therapy with nebulized distilled water or 10% NaCl will result in adequate specimens in 90% of cases.
B. The presence of acid-fast bacilli in gastric washings is diagnostic of mycobacterial disease.
C. Sputum induction is most commonly used to diagnose tuberculosis or lung malignancy.
D. Gastric lavage is most useful late in the day after the patient has been awake and swallowing secretions.

Question 5.5. **Which of the following statements is/are correct regarding occupational and environmental exposure history in patients with lung disease?**

A. Passive smoking has been shown to increase the incidence of respiratory infections.

B. Occupational exposures up to 25 years prior to presentation may be useful in evaluating lung disease.

C. Family history is often useful in cases of exposure and infectious illnesses.

D. Toxic exposures other than inhalation injuries may be related to the lungs.

Question 5.6.   Match the lung sounds to the appropriate description:

1. Fine crackles
2. Coarse crackles
3. Wheezes
4. Rhonchi

A. Continuous and low-pitched: occur mainly in large airways.

B. Discontinuous, high-pitched, short duration; usually caused by small airway closure.

C. Discontinuous, low-pitched, and long duration; associated with bronchitis or bronchopneumonia.

D. Continuous and high-pitched; usually occur in the presence of bronchospasm.

Question 5.7.   Match the clinical condition to the characteristic pulse with which it is associated.

1. Status asthmaticus
2. Hypovolemic shock
3. Sepsis
4. Myocardial infarction with decreased left ventricular function

A. Weak, thready pulse

B. Bounding pulse

C. Every other pulsation is weak

D. Decline in pulse pressure during inspiration

Question 5.8.   Match the following conditions to the potential physical findings seen on routine inspection and examination:

1. Lung abscess
2. Sarcoidosis
3. Asthma treated with inhaled steroids
4. Nasal polyps

A. Paralysis of the face on one side

B. Oral thrush

C. Poor dental hygiene and foul-smelling breath.

D. Allergic rhinitis

Question 5.9.   Match the clinical picture with the sputum character:

1. Viral pneumonia
2. Pneumococcal lobar pneumonia
3. Recent asthma exacerbation
4. Tuberculosis
5. Lung abscess

A. Scant sputum composed of mucous mixed with blood ("rusty"), later becoming purulent.

B. Expectoration of large volumes of yellow or green sputum that is foul-smelling.

C. Scant mucoid sputum initially with a few streaks of blood, may later become purulent.

D. Sputum is thick and tenacious and contains bronchial mucus plugs.
E. Chronic production of mucoid sputum associated with blood streaking.

Question 5.10. **Determine whether the given statements apply to:**

A. Lateral or chest wall pain, or
B. Central or visceral chest pain

1. Pain which arises in internal organs and is conducted through afferent fibers of the vagus nerve.
2. Pain that is conducted through the intercostal and phrenic nerves.
3. Occurs with neoplasms of the major bronchi or mediastinum.
4. Pain that is sharp, well-localized, and increased with breathing.
5. Pain associated with trauma to the chest wall.

Question 5.11. **True/False. Under the following conditions an examiner would expect the chest to be dull to percussion:**

A. Pneumothorax
B. Pleural effusion
C. Atelectasis
D. Hyperinflation
E. Pneumonic consolidation

Question 5.12. **The following statements are TRUE/FALSE regarding the presence of coughing:**

A. Cough receptors are located in the large bronchi, trachea, and larynx.
B. Irritation of cough receptors occurs only in the presence of abnormal respiratory secretions.
C. Most acute and self-limiting coughs are secondary to a viral respiratory infection.
D. Patients with asthma may present with the sole complaint of coughing.
E. Cough may occur as a side effect of β-adrenergic blocking agents or angiotensin converting enzyme (ACE) inhibiting drugs.

Question 5.13. **Which of the following conditions is NOT associated with Horner's syndrome?**

A. Loss of sweating
B. Meiosis
C. Facial muscle atrophy
D. Ipsilateral enophthalmos

ANSWERS

Answer 5.1. **A, B, C**

A wide variety of physical findings outside the thorax may occur in patients with pulmonary disease. Hypoxemia is associated with cyanosis if 5 g/dl or more of reduced hemoglobin is present in the capillary blood. Central cyanosis implies involvement of gas transfer in the lungs and affects the tongue as well as the extremities. Peripheral cyanosis without central cyanosis implies a circulatory problem such as vascular spasm or shock. Clubbing is seen with many chest diseases, such as neoplasms, bronchiectasis, and lung abscess; it may also be inherited as a familial trait or may occur with diseases of other organs such as the liver.

Reference: page 89

Answer 5.2.   **A, B, C**

A pleural friction rub is a grating sound associated with breathing. Rapid tape record-ings have demonstrated that pleural rubs are actually a series of small explosions, just as crackles are. Pleural friction rubs are generally loud and sound as if they are imme-diately below the stethoscope. They occur during both inspiration and expiration. The rub will often occur simultaneously with the patient's chest pain.

Reference: page 89

Answer 5.3.   **All are correct**

The term hemoptysis means coughing of blood. It is important to determine the dura-tion and to note whether there is gross blood, blood-tinged sputum, or blood-streaked sputum. Attempts should be made to determine the amount of blood produced and whether it is bright red or dark and whether or not it contains clots. Hematemesis, or vomiting of blood, may be confused with hemoptysis. Hematemesis more often pro-duces dark red blood that is usually acid, while hemoptysis is alkaline. With he-matemesis blood streaking of sputum is unusual, while with hemoptysis it is common. Vomited blood frequently contains food particles, while this is rare with hemoptysis. While the majority of episodes of hemoptysis in earlier years were due to bronchiecta-sis, tuberculosis, or unknown causes, in more recent reports (following the appearance of fiberoptic bronchoscopy), the most common cause of hemoptysis is chronic bronchi-tis. One-third of cases are still due to unknown causes.

Reference: pages 85–86

Answer 5.4.   **A, C**

If a patient is unable to produce sputum, inhalation of a nebulized solution of 3 or 4 ml distilled water or 10% sodium chloride results in the induction of an adequate specimen for examination in over 90% of cases. The procedure is most often used for patients sus-pected of having tuberculosis or a lung malignancy, and to search for *Pneumocystis carinii* infection in patients with AIDS. The usefulness of gastric washings is based on the fact that most coughed secretions are swallowed rather than expectorated. The pro-cedure is performed immediately upon awakening, before the stomach has emptied. The presence of acid-fast bacilli on smears of gastric washings is not diagnostic of my-cobacterial disease, because saprophytic mycobacteria are often present in the stomach. Mycobacterial culture is required to confirm the presence of pathogens.

Reference: page 85

Answer 5.5.   **All are correct**

Passive exposure to cigarette smoke in the home or the workplace is an increasingly rec-ognized cause of respiratory symptoms in children whose parents smoke, and passive smoking has been shown to increase the incidence of respiratory infections. Occupa-tional exposures may have occurred many years before presentation; exposure to as-bestos may result in the development of a pleural mesothelioma 25 years or more after the exposure has ceased. Family history is useful in recognizing inherited disorders (cystic fibrosis, α_1-antitrypsin deficiency), asthma or allergy history, or infectious dis-eases, such as tuberculosis or viral respiratory diseases, that are often spread by house-hold contact.

Reference: page 82

Answer 5.6. **1-B; 2-C; 3-D; 4-A**

Robertson and Coope introduced the term "crackles" to describe the series of tiny explosions heard over the chest wall during inspiration (discontinuous). Early fine crackles are usually heard with small airway closure at end-expiration and disappear after a few breaths. Coarse, early inspiratory crackles are associated with bronchitis or bronchopneumonia. Continuous breath sounds are either wheezes, which are high-pitched and arise in small airways, or rhonchi, which are low-pitched and occur in large airways. Wheezes generally occur in the presence of bronchospasm and are an important finding in asthma. Rhonchi are common in severely ill patients whose secretions have collected in proximal airways.

Reference: pages 88–89

Answer 5.7. **1-D; 2-A; 3-B; 4-C**

Peripheral pulses may be useful in the monitoring of patients. A weak, thready pulse indicates a low cardiac stroke volume, as seen in cardiogenic or hypovolemic shock. A bounding pulse is common in sepsis associated with low vascular resistance and a high cardiac output. Pulsus alternans (every other pulse is weak) is associated with severely depressed left ventricular function. Pulsus paradoxus (a decline in systolic blood pressure greater than 10 mm Hg during inspiration) is present in patients with severe airways obstruction (as in status asthmaticus), as well as those with pericardial tamponade.

Reference: page 90

Answer 5.8. **1-C; 2-A; 3-B; 4-D**

Patients with lung abscess or empyema frequently have foul-smelling breath and poor dental hygiene, and may have trouble swallowing. Sarcoidosis may involve the salivary and lacrimal glands, with dryness of the oral mucosa and conjunctivae; involvement of the parotid gland may be associated with paralysis of the facial nerve (Bell's palsy). Oropharyngeal candidiasis (thrush) may be associated with inhaled steroids or antibiotic therapy and is also common in immunosuppressed patients. Nasal polyps occur with respiratory allergies and may cause epistaxis.

Reference: page 86

Answer 5.9. **1-C; 2-A; 3-D; 4-E; 5-B**

Viral infections of the lower respiratory tract are associated at first with scant mucoid sputum, which may contain a few streaks of blood. Later the sputum may become copious and purulent with or without bacterial superinfection. In pneumococcal lobar pneumonia the sputum is usually scanty and composed of mucus tinged with blood ("rusty"); later, sputum may become purulent. Asthmatics who are recovering from an acute attack usually produce sputum that is thick and tenacious and contains bronchial mucus plugs. Tuberculosis is associated most often with the chronic production of mucoid sputum that may be associated with blood streaking. Lung abscesses are associated with expectoration of large volumes of yellow or green sputum, the colors being produced by pigments released from degenerating neutrophils. Approximately 60% of patients with lung abscess will have foul-smelling sputum associated with bad breath, anorexia, and weight loss.

Reference: pages 84–85

Answer 5.10.   **1-B; 2-A; 3-B; 4-A; 5-A**

There are two basic types of chest pain: that which arises in the chest wall structures and is conducted through the intercostal and phrenic nerves (lateral or chest wall pain) and that which arises in the internal organs and is conducted through the afferent fibers of the vagus nerve (central or visceral pain). Visceral chest pain occurs with neoplasms of the major bronchi and mediastinum; abnormalities of the heart, aorta, and pericardium; or diseases that cause esophageal pain. Chest wall pain is sharp, often well localized, and is increased by deep breathing or coughing (pleuritic pain or pleurisy). Pleuritic pain is associated with any disease that causes inflammation of the parietal pleura, such as infections, trauma, or tumors.

Reference: page 83

Answer 5.11.   **B, C, E - True; A, D - False**

Percussion of the chest is useful because the chest contains structures of both air and fluid density, and in the presence of disease their relationships may vary. With pleural effusions, consolidations, large intrathoracic masses, or atelectasis, the chest is dull to percussion. With pneumothorax or hyperinflation, the chest is hyperresonant.

Reference: page 87

Answer 5.12.   **A, C, D, E - True; B - False**

Cough receptors are located in the large bronchi, trachea, and larynx and respond to respiratory secretions in the large airways. However, irritation of the cough receptors may occur in the absence of abnormal secretions, as with inhalation of toxic fumes or a mild asthma attack. Most acute and self-limiting coughs are secondary to a viral respiratory infection, while chronic and persistent coughs are most often associated with chronic bronchitis or postnasal drip. Cough may be the sole complaint in patients with mild asthma. Cough with or without bronchospasm may occur as a side effect of β-adrenergic antagonists as well as the ACE inhibiting drugs.

Reference: page 84

Answer 5.13.   **C**

Patients who have pulmonary neoplasms may have one of several paraneoplastic syndromes, which are usually related to invasion of the tumor cells or production of hormones by tumor cells. Horner's syndrome occurs when apical lung tumors invade outside the pleura and into the superior cervical ganglion. There is ipsilateral enophthalmos, loss of sweating, and meiosis (the triad of ptosis, meiosis, and anhydrosis).

Reference: page 89

chapter 6

Invasive Diagnostic Procedures

QUESTIONS

Question 6.1. **Concerning thoracentesis, which of the following statements is true?**

A. Ten millimeters of pleural fluid on a lateral decubitus chest film (as measured from the inner border of the rib to the lower part of the lung), indicate enough fluid is present for a diagnostic thoracentesis.
B. The gross appearance of pleural fluid provides little useful clinical information.
C. Blood-tinged pleural fluid implies the presence of at least 100,000 RBCs per cubic millimeter.
D. Blood-tinged fluid indicates the presence of trauma, malignancy, or pulmonary embolus, as the cause of the effusion.

Question 6.2. **A 30-year-old man presents to the emergency room with acute onset of dyspnea, tachycardia, and tachypnea. Decreased breath sounds are heard over the posterior right hemithorax, with dullness to percussion. Upright chest film reveals a moderate right pleural effusion. Regarding this patient's diagnosis, which of the following statements is true?**

A. Gross blood found on thoracentesis indicates the presence of a hemothorax, consistent with trauma, malignancy, or pulmonary infarction.
B. Milky-white pleural fluid indicates the presence of a chylous effusion.
C. A pleural fluid triglyceride level in the normal range, with an elevated cholesterol level is consistent with a chylous effusion.
D. An exudative pleural effusion with a lymphocytosis on cell differential is an indication for a pleural biopsy (provided pleural fluid studies are nondiagnostic).

Question 6.3. **Concerning exudative pleural effusions, which of the following statements is false?**

A. In parapneumonic effusions, a pH ≤7.0 suggests a complicated or loculated effusion, which may progress to an empyema.
B. In contrast to low pleural fluid pH, pleural fluid glucose is usually normal in complicated parapneumonic effusions.
C. Lymphocytosis on pleural fluid differential cell count suggests malignancy or tuberculosis as the cause of the effusion.
D. Adenosine deaminase levels of pleural fluid are often elevated in tuberculous effusions.

Question 6.4. **A 36-year-old woman is suspected of having sarcoidosis. Chest film reveals a bilaterally symmetrical interstitial infiltrate. Which of the following statements is/are true concerning bronchoscopy?**

A. Non-caseating granulomas are identified in up to 90% of sarcoid patients, when a minimum of four transbronchial biopsies are submitted.
B. Increasing the number of biopsy specimens can increase the diagnostic yield to approximately 95%, even in patients with no radiographic evidence of disease.
C. A T-lymphocyte CD4:CD8 ratio of 1:10 is consistent with a diagnosis of sarcoidosis.
D. Open lung biopsy should be considered in the absence of granulomas, pathogenic organisms, or malignancy from fiberoptic bronchoscopy.

Question 6.5. **A 68-year-old white man presents with a large left pleural effusion. Diagnostic thoracentesis yields straw colored fluid, with an LDH of 663 U/liter, protein of 5.9 g/dl, and 2080 nucleated cells/mm³ with a lymphocyte predominance. Concerning this patient, which of the following statements is/are true?**

A. In malignant pleural effusions, initial pleural fluid cytologic exam is diagnostic approximately 60% of the time.
B. The presence of mesothelial cells in the pleural fluid is evidence that the patient does not have tuberculosis.
C. If the pleural fluid is nondiagnostic, a pleural biopsy is indicated, with specimens sent for pathology, acid-fast bacilli culture, and fungal studies.
D. Elevated pleural fluid amylase indicates either esophageal rupture, pancreatitis, or malignancy, and isoenzymes of amylase may be helpful in determining which is the cause.

Question 6.6. **Regarding fiberoptic bronchoscopy, which of the following statements is/are correct?**

A. Biopsies of visible endobronchial carcinomas are diagnostic in approximately 70% of cases.
B. Biopsy yield of nonvisible lesions depends on tumor location and size on chest radiograph.
C. By combining brushings, transbronchial biopsies, and washings, the diagnostic yield of nonvisible peripheral lesions is approximately 10%.
D. Biopsy yield of nonvisible hilar lesions is approximately 90%.

Question 6.7. **Regarding flexible fiberoptic bronchoscopy, which of the following statements is/are correct?**

A. Common complications include hypoxemia, bleeding, cardiac arrhythmias, bronchospasm, pneumonia, and pneumothorax.
B. Fever is reported in over 60% of patients within 24 hours postbronchoscopy.
C. Uremia creates a major risk of bleeding, with 45% of uremic patients having significant bleeding with transbronchial biopsy.
D. Fiberoptic bronchoscopy produces an average decline in PaO_2 of 15 to 20 mm Hg, which is prevented by intubation and mechanical ventilation.

Question 6.8. **Regarding bronchoalveolar lavage (BAL), which of the following statements is/are correct?**

A. The technique involves instillation of an aliquot of sterile saline through the bronchoscope, followed by syringe aspiration or gravity drainage, with recovery of approximately 60% of the instilled volume.
B. BAL fluid from AIDS patients revealing *Pneumocystis carinii, Legionella, Histoplasma,* or respiratory syncytial virus confirms the presence of a pulmonary infection with these organisms.

C. BAL findings of milky or opaque lavage fluid, large cellular eosinophilic bodies, and proteinaceous staining material, establish a diagnosis of alveolar proteinosis.
D. Isolation of cytomegalovirus (CMV) or herpes simplex virus (HSV) in AIDS patients by BAL is diagnostic of infection with these organisms.

Question 6.9. **A 40-year-old man is intubated and mechanically ventilated. A chest radiograph reveals a right lower lobe infiltrate. Regarding this patient, which of the following statements is/are correct?**

A. Protected specimen brush (PSB) culture results are diagnostic of an infectious etiology regardless of the concomitant use of antibiotics.
B. Transbronchial needle aspiration is of limited use in diagnosing an infectious etiology in this patient.
C. One hundred colony forming units (CFUs) per milliliter of inoculated saline via PSB is adequate to ensure an accurate diagnosis.
D. Transthoracic needle aspiration may be beneficial in determining a specific infectious etiology, but this patient is at an increased risk for pneumothorax.

Question 6.10. **Video-assisted thoracic surgery (VATS) is becoming more useful in the therapy of chest diseases. Concerning VATS, which of the following statements is/are correct?**

A. Complication rate of thoracoscopy is about 10%, and includes prolonged air leak, wound infection, and bleeding requiring transfusion or reoperation.
B. In undiagnosed exudative pleural effusions (after thoracentesis and pleural biopsy), VATS offers no more diagnostic benefit than a repeat pleural biopsy.
C. VATS provides a less invasive means of diagnosing of solitary peripheral nodules and in the treatment of bronchopleural fistula, when compared to thoracotomy.
D. VATS is often used as an initial diagnostic tool in evaluating patients with pleural effusions.

ANSWERS

Answer 6.1. **A**

The gross appearance of pleural fluid is often useful, especially in cases of hemothorax, chylothorax, chyliform effusion, or empyema. Blood-tinged fluid requires the presence of at least 5000 RBCs/mm³, while grossly bloody effusions are seen with 100,000 RBCs/mm³ or more. Pleural fluid hematocrit should be measured on all grossly bloody effusions to determine the presence or absence of a hemothorax, which requires the pleural fluid hematocrit to be at least 50% that of peripheral blood. Over 15% of transudates and 40% of exudates are blood-tinged, providing little clinical relevance.

Reference: pages 92–94

Answer 6.2. **D**

A hemothorax is present when the pleural fluid hematocrit is 50% or more of peripheral blood. Milky-white effusions may be seen with chylous effusions, chyliform effusions, or empyema. Chylous effusions have an elevated triglyceride level, while chyliform effusions have an elevated cholesterol level, and are seen with long-standing effusions of various causes. A lymphocytic exudative effusion is an indication for repeat thoracentesis with pleural biopsy, unless the original thoracentesis is diagnostic.

Reference: pages 93–94

Answer 6.3. **B**

A low pleural fluid pH indicates a complicated effusion in patients with parapneumonic effusions. Pleural fluid glucose is usually concomitantly decreased with pH in patients with complicated parapneumonic effusions. Pleural fluid lymphocytosis is most commonly associated with granulomatous or malignant pleuritis. A pleural fluid adenosine deaminase (ADA) level less than 50 U/liter is evidence against pleural tuberculosis.

Reference: pages 94–95

Answer 6.4. **A, B, D - True; C - False**

Transbronchial biopsy is the biopsy procedure of choice in diagnosing sarcoidosis, and is positive in 90% or more of cases when adequate samples are obtained. CD4:CD8 ratios are helpful in bronchoalveolar lavage, especially in separating hypersensitivity pneumonitis from sarcoidosis. The ratio in sarcoidosis is usually 20:1, while hypersensitivity pneumonitis is much lower. Open lung biopsy, usually via thoracoscopy or mediastinotomy, is indicated in the rare case where less invasive procedures fail and a diagnosis is required.

Reference: page 98

Answer 6.5. **All are correct**

Elevated pleural fluid amylase is seen in esophageal rupture, malignancy, or pancreatic effusions. Esophageal rupture and malignancy may show elevated salivary amylase while pancreatic effusions reveal elevated pancreatic amylase. Most malignancies causing elevated amylase levels are adenocarcinomas.

Reference: pages 94–95

Answer 6.6. **B, D**

Biopsies of visible lesions are diagnostic for malignancy in over 90% of cases. Nonvisible lesions have a variable success depending on tumor size and location, with hilar lesions having a 90% success rate, while peripheral lesions have a 36% success when brush, biopsy, and washings are combined.

Reference: page 97

Answer 6.7. **A, C**

Fever occurs in up to 16% of postbronchoscopy patients. Uremia, platelet dysfunction, coagulopathies, drugs, immunosuppression, and malignancy all increase the risk of bleeding with transbronchial biopsy. Fiberoptic bronchoscopy produces a 15–20 mm Hg decline in PaO_2, in ventilated and nonventilated patients alike.

Reference: pages 100–101

Answer 6.8. **A, B, C**

BAL, when properly performed, can be diagnostic in many disease processes. The finding of CMV and HSV in lavage fluid is not diagnostic however, because these organisms are frequently colonizers of the upper respiratory tract in immunodeficient patients. The characteristics of BAL fluid in patients with alveolar proteinosis are helpful in establishing the diagnosis. Isolation of respiratory pathogens is an important indication for BAL in patients with AIDS.

Reference: pages 101–102

Answer 6.9.   **B, D**

PSB is a very useful diagnostic tool when performed properly, and is especially helpful in nonintubated patients who are not on antibiotics. The significance of positive PSB cultures in mechanically ventilated patients on antibiotics has not been established. Transbronchial needle aspiration is useful to diagnose malignancy, and transthoracic needle aspiration may be helpful in diagnosing infectious etiology. PSB must yield a minimum of 10^4 CFUs/ml of inoculated saline in order to be considered positive in most reported series.

Reference: pages 102—103

Answer 6.10.   **A, C**

Although VATS is becoming much more useful in the management of chest diseases, thoracentesis and pleural biopsy remain the initial diagnostic procedures for patients with significant pleural effusions. Thoracoscopy is indicated when less invasive studies are nondiagnostic. Importannt uses of thoracoscopy include biopsy of peripheral lung lesions, mediastinal lymph node biopsy, therapy of bronchopleural fistula, and pleurodesis.

Reference: pages 104–106

chapter 7

Chest Imaging

QUESTIONS

Question 7.1. **Which of the following statements is/are correct regarding routine screening with chest radiographs?**

A. Routine screening is not necessary in patients under 20 years of age.
B. Lateral views are not necessary in patients 20–39 years of age.
C. Lateral views should be used as part of normal screening in patients 40 years of age or older.
D. Lateral films should be obtained whenever chest disease is suspected.

Question 7.2. **Which of the following structures contribute(s) significantly to the normal hilar shadows on normal chest radiographs?**

A. Pulmonary arteries
B. Lower lobe pulmonary veins
C. Upper lobe pulmonary veins
D. Major bronchi

Question 7.3. **For which of the following reason(s) is fluoroscopy of the chest *NOT* acceptable as a screening procedure?**

A. Increased x-ray exposure
B. Small lesions are often overlooked
C. No permanent records of the exam are available
D. Fluoroscopy provides little improvement over routine PA and lateral views when evaluating pulmonary nodules.

Question 7.4. **Under which of the following condition(s) would magnetic resonance imaging (MRI) have diagnostic advantage over computed tomography (CT) as the initial procedure of choice?**

A. Interstitial lung disease
B. Superior sulcus tumors
C. Aortic dissection
D. Paracardiac masses

Question 7.5. **Which of the following statements is/are correct regarding the use of ultrasound in detecting thoracic disease?**

A. Ultrasound has limited usefulness in evaluation of the lung parenchyma.
B. Ultrasound is the procedure of choice to detect or exclude pericardial effusions.
C. Ultrasound is useful in obtaining information concerning valvular heart disease.
D. Ultrasound should be routinely use to localize pleural effusions prior to drainage.

Question 7.6. **Which of the following conditions may be indications for pulmonary angiography?**

A. Hypoplasia of the pulmonary artery
B. Suspected pulmonary arteriovenous malformation
C. Anomalous pulmonary venous drainage
D. Pulmonary thromboembolism

Question 7.7. Determine whether the following statements are TRUE or FALSE regarding the radiographic anatomy of the airways.

A. Deviation of the trachea to the right may be a normal finding.
B. The course of the left mainstem bronchus is more vertical than that of the right mainstem bronchus.
C. The left mainstem bronchus is larger in both length and transverse diameter than the right mainstem bronchus.
D. Most radiographic presentations of atelectasis are lobar in distribution.

Question 7.8. Determine if the following statements are TRUE or FALSE concerning the pulmonary vascular system.

A. The main pulmonary artery and its bifurcation lie entirely within the pericardial sac.
B. The pulmonary arteries lie posterior to their respective main bronchi in the hila.
C. Pulmonary artery hypertension is usually associated with enlargement of the right descending pulmonary artery.
D. It is easier to identify the pulmonary veins in the lower lung fields than in the upper lung fields.

Question 7.9. Which of the following segments of the lung is NOT a frequent site for aspiration?

A. Posterior segment of the right upper lobe
B. Superior segment of the right lower lobe
C. Apical-posterior segment of the left upper lobe
D. Posterior basal segment of the left lower lobe

Question 7.10. Which of the following statements is NOT correct regarding the use of ventilation-perfusion lung scanning?

A. Its major indication is in the investigation of pulmonary thromboembolism.
B. The absence of perfusion to an entire lobe is specific for thromboembolic disease.
C. Perfusion studies are diagnostically valuable only when the scan image is normal or can be compared with a current chest radiograph and ventilation scan.
D. Lung scans are useful in evaluating preoperative lung function.

Question 7.11. Match the chest abnormality with the type of erect chest radiograph view which would be most useful to demonstrate it.

1. Free pleural fluid
2. Pleural plaques due to asbestosis
3. Lingular lobe collapse
4. Small pneumothorax

A. Lordotic view
B. Expiration film
C. Lateral decubitus view
D. Oblique views

ANSWERS

Answer 7.1.   **All are correct**

Studies done by Sagel et al. of over 100,000 chest radiographs of a hospital-based population concluded that routine screening examinations, obtained solely because of hospital admission or scheduled surgery, are not warranted in patients under 20, and that the lateral projection can be safely eliminated from routine screening examination in patients 20–39 years of age. A lateral film should be obtained whenever chest disease is suspected and in screening examination of patients 40 years of age or older.

Reference: page 112

Answer 7.2.   **A, C**

The hila are composed of the pulmonary arteries and their main branches, the upper lobe pulmonary veins, the major bronchi, and the lymph nodes. The lower lobe pulmonary veins do not cross the hila and therefore do not contribute to the hilar shadows. The bronchi account for little of the hilar opacity, since they are filled with air, and normally lymph nodes are too small to add to the size or density. Therefore, normal hilar shadows consist mostly of the large pulmonary arteries and upper lobe veins.

Reference: page 115

Answer 7.3.   **A, B, C**

In past years, fluoroscopy of the chest was used as a screening procedure for routine chest examination. This no longer acceptable because: (a) the patient's exposure to x-rays is much greater even during a short fluoroscopic examination than during standard radiographs; (b) small lesions in the lung fields are overlooked at fluoroscopy; and (c) usually no permanent record of the fluoroscopic examination is available. Chest fluoroscopy can be useful when trying to determine if a suspected pulmonary nodule on a chest radiograph (a) is real versus a superimposition of unrelated shadows or (b) is intrapulmonary versus extrapulmonary. Rarely, arteriovenous aneurysms presenting as pulmonary nodules may be seen to pulsate at fluoroscopy.

Reference: pages 120–121

Answer 7.4.   **B, D**

CT has application in vascular imaging in the thorax, most notably for suspected aortic dissection. High-resolution CT of the lung parenchyma has been developed in the last few years and has become widely useful for evaluating interstitial lung disease. There are a few conditions in which MRI has a real diagnostic advantage over CT; these include superior sulcus tumors, upper extremity deep vein thrombosis, and cardiac and paracardiac masses.

Reference: pages 121–123

Answer 7.5.   **A, B, C**

Ultrasound has limited usefulness in evaluating the lungs, since the sound beam is transmitted poorly by the air-containing alveoli and airways. Ultrasound is widely used to evaluate disorders of the heart and aortic root, and is the procedure of choice to detect or exclude pericardial effusions. Unique information can also be obtained concerning valvular heart disease such as mitral stenosis, the presence of vegetations or clots in the cardiac chambers, and global or segmental abnormalities of cardiac contraction. Ultrasound is also useful in precisely locating pleural effusions for aspiration and drainage. It should be emphasized that ultrasound should not be used routinely for this purpose, because most effusions can be safely and easily aspirated after localization by chest film and physical examination.

Reference: page 125

Answer 7.6. A, B, C, D

Pulmonary angiography involves the rapid injection of a radiopaque dye into the pulmonary circulation. Angiography is principally useful for investigating pulmonary thromboembolic disease, and is almost always indicated when a massive pulmonary embolus is suspected as the basis for circulatory collapse. Less common indications for angiography include (*a*) suspected congenital abnormalities of the arterial system, such as agenesis or hypoplasia of a pulmonary artery; (*b*) suspected congenital abnormalities of the pulmonary venous circulation, such as anomalous pulmonary venous drainage and pulmonary varix; and (*c*) suspected pulmonary A-V malformations.

Reference: pages 126–127

Answer 7.7. A, D - True; B, C - False

The trachea is a midline structure; however, a slight deviation to the right after entering the thorax is a normal finding due to the position of the aortic arch and should not be misinterpreted as evidence of displacement. The trachea divides into the two major bronchi at the carina. The course of the right mainstem bronchus distally is more vertical than that of the left. The transverse diameter of the right main bronchus at total lung capacity is greater than that of the left (average 15.3 mm versus 13.0 mm in adults), although its length before origin of the upper lobe bronchus as measured at necropsy is shorter (average 2.2 cm compared to 5 cm on the left). Lobar consolidation of the lung is frequently associated with loss of volume (atelectasis). However, atelectasis of pulmonary segments occurs less often because collapse is prevented by collateral air drift; thus, most radiographic presentations of atelectasis are lobar.

Reference: page 114

Answer 7.8. A, C, D - True; B - False

The main pulmonary artery is 4–5 cm in length and about 3 cm in diameter in adults. It lies entirely within the pericardial sac, as does its bifurcation. The right pulmonary artery lies posterior to the aorta and the superior vena cava and anterior to the right main bronchus. The left pulmonary artery divides within the left hilum after passing immediately anterior and laterally to the lower portion of the left main bronchus. Radiographic measurement of a segment of the pulmonary vascular tree may provide useful information. Pulmonary artery hypertension is generally associated with enlargement of the right descending pulmonary artery.

Reference: pages 115–116

Answer 7.9. C

Of clinical significance is the fact that several segmental bronchi are located posteriorly, which renders them frequent recipients of aspirated material when in the supine position, and are likely sites for the development of aspiration pneumonia. The dorsally located segments that are frequent sites for aspiration include the posterior segment of the right upper lobe; the posterior basal and superior segments of the right lower lobe; and the posterior basal and superior segments of the left lower lobe.

Reference: page 114

Answer 7.10.   **B**

The major indication for lung scanning is the investigation of pulmonary thromboembolism. Perfusion studies are diagnostically valuable only when the scan image is normal or can be compared with a current chest radiograph and ventilation scan. The absence of perfusion in an area of lung is nonspecific. It can be due to thromboembolic disease or to primary pulmonary vascular disease such as arteritis; it can be secondary to airway obstruction or other abnormalities of ventilation; or it can result from destruction of lung parenchyma, as in bullous emphysema. Prior to surgery, a lung scan can determine the contribution to overall pulmonary function of the region of the lung to be resected.

Reference: page 129

Answer 7.11.   **1 - C; 2 - D; 3 - A; 4 - B**

The lateral decubitus film is useful for demonstrating a small amount of free pleural fluid, particularly if blunting of a costophrenic sulcus is present on routine PA films. Some reports have emphasized the value of oblique chest radiographs in detecting pleural plaques due to asbestosis. The lordotic view is useful for recognizing collapse of the lingula or right middle lobe when these areas become very thin and cast minimal shadows on the PA film. A small pneumothorax is often difficult to see on a routine PA inspiratory film. On expiration, the volume of the thorax and of the lungs within it is reduced, but the amount of air in the pleural sac remains essentially unchanged. The pneumothorax then occupies a larger percentage of the area of the thorax and is more easily visible.

Reference: pages 117–118

chapter 8

Clinical Pulmonary Function Testing, Exercise Testing, and Disability Evaluation

---

QUESTIONS

Question 8.1. **Concerning spirometry, which of the following statements is/are correct?**

A. The measurements of $FEV_{0.5}$, FEV_1, and FEV_3 are not altered by a decrease in total lung capacity (TLC).
B. The ratio of FEV_1/FVC is a sensitive means of evaluating airway obstruction, and is independent of patient size.
C. The FEV_1/FVC ratio is generally not specific for airway obstruction if the patient has concomitant restrictive lung disease.
D. A reduction in FEV_3/FVC ratio is evidence of long-standing obstructive ventilatory impairment.

Question 8.2. **Spirometric indices provide information regarding airway obstruction and restriction. Regarding spirometry, which of the following statements is correct?**

A. Forced expiratory flows (FEFs), such as $FEF_{25-75}\%$ and $FEF_{200-1200}$, are average flow rates (as measured by volume change over time change) and are easily reproducible in normal subjects.
B. For valid results, the largest FVC and second-largest FVC should vary by a maximum of 5% or 100 cc, whichever is greater.
C. The FEV_1 and FVC should be recorded from the same curve of multiple attempts.
D. A single, well performed FVC maneuver is adequate to ensure valid test results.

Question 8.3. **Regarding flow-volume curves, determine whether the following statements are true or false:**

A. The peak of the curve on the y-axis is equivalent to the FVC of a spirogram.
B. The latter two-thirds of the exhalation curve is relatively effort dependent.
C. Early in the development of obstructive airway disease, expiratory flow at low lung volumes is decreased but the volume exhaled is normal, causing a characteristic appearance of the flow-volume loop.
D. The flow-volume loop is not helpful in patients with restrictive ventilatory impairment.

Question 8.4. **Which of the following statements concerning pulmonary function tests are true or false?**

A. Peak expiratory flow is the highest flow rate that occurs during a forced exhalation during tidal breathing.

B. The portability of peak expiratory flow meters make them very useful in home monitoring of airway obstruction, in patients with asthma.

C. Bronchoprovocation tests are considered diagnostic of airway hyperresponsiveness when the dose of histamine or methacholine which causes a 10% fall in FEV_1 is 8.0 micromoles or less.

D. Cigarette smoking in patients with obstructive airways disease causes a desensitization to bronchoprovocation testing, indicating a decreased airway hyperresponsiveness in this patient group.

Question 8.5. Regarding determination of lung volumes, which of the following statements is/are correct?

A. The closed circuit helium dilution method of determination of functional residual capacity (FRC) adequately measures FRC, including the volume of gas within lung bullae.

B. Accuracy of the gas dilution techniques to measure lung volumes is dependent on beginning and ending the test at a volume other than residual volume (RV).

C. Plethysmographic techniques for determining lung volumes measure both the communicating and noncommunicating compartments, while gas dilution methods determine only communicating FRC or RV.

D. Plethysmographic determination of lung volumes is accurate regardless of starting volume.

Question 8.6. Determine which of the following statements concerning lung mechanics are true or false?

A. Static lung compliance (CLST) decreases with age.

B. Airway resistance (R_{AW}) should be measured at low flow rates to avoid the effects of dynamic compression of the airways.

C. Alveolar filling diseases cause a decreased static lung compliance.

D. Total lung compliance is independent of chest wall compliance (CWST).

Question 8.7. Regarding diffusion capacity for carbon monoxide (DLCO), which of the following statements is/are correct?

A. The single-breath method is the DLCO method most sensitive to ventilation-perfusion abnormalities.

B. The major resistance to the diffusion of CO from the alveoli to the blood is the state of the alveolar-capillary membrane, with pulmonary capillary hemoglobin playing a negligible role.

C. Measured DLCO is significantly dependent on the available surface area for gas exchange.

D. Anemia alone can cause a reduction in the measurement of DLCO, despite normal lungs.

Question 8.8. Regarding exercise and exercise testing, determine which of the following statements are true or false:

A. The best metabolic index of the work capacity in a given individual is the anaerobic threshold (AT).

B. Estimation of an individual's VO_2 from nomograms based on weight and treadmill speed and inclination does not account for the contribution of anaerobic metabolism to VO_2.

C. The cardiac output is the limiting factor for $VO_{2\,max}$ in normal subjects.

D. The linear increase in cardiac output with exercise is primarily due to increased stroke volume in normal subjects.

Question 8.9.   Which of the following statements is/are correct regarding exercise physiology and ventilation?

A. Normal individuals are able to maintain minute ventilation above 60% of their maximum voluntary ventilation (MVV), while patients with moderate to severe lung disease are unable to sustain minute ventilation above 60% of their MVV.
B. Patients with lung disease have reduced ventilatory reserves and increased ventilatory requirements for a given level of exercise.
C. During exercise, dead space ventilation (VD/VT) decreases in normal subjects but is unchanged in patients with COPD.
D. The ventilatory equivalent for CO_2 (VE/VCO_2) is a measure of the efficiency of CO_2 elimination, and is usually elevated in patients with COPD.

Question 8.10.   Exercise training produces all of the following effects EXCEPT:

A. Maximum cardiac output increases via an increase in the maximum stroke volume.
B. There is a higher distribution of the cardiac output to exercising muscles, increasing oxidative capacity, mitochondrial activity, and enhancing enzymes to promote the use of free fatty acids.
C. Endurance training in COPD patients does not result in an increase in mitochondrial enzyme activities as it does in normal subjects.
D. VO_{2max} in deconditioned patients with COPD increases an average of 40% during a well-supervised training program.

ANSWERS

Answer 8.1.   **B**

Simple spirometry involves forceful exhalation from total lung capacity (TLC), of a volume of air as measured over time. The curve created provides evidence of airway obstruction and/or restriction, when compared to normal controls. The $FEV_{0.5}$, FEV_1, and FEV_3, are volumes of exhaled air as measured over the initial 0.5, 1.0, and 3.0 seconds, respectively. All are decreased by any process that inhibits expiratory flow, a reduced effort, or a reduced TLC. The ratio of the forced expiratory volume divided by the forced vital capacity (FEV_1/FVC), provides a more sensitive means of evaluating obstruction to flow, and is relatively independent of patient size. The FEV_1/FVC is a specific measure of airway obstruction with or without associated restrictive lung disease. The FEV_3/FVC includes flow at relatively low lung values, when flow rates are reduced early in obstructive disease states.

Reference: page 133

Answer 8.2.   **B**

Forced expiratory flows are measured graphically by dividing the volume change by the time required to make that change. The commonly reported FEFs include $FEF_{25-75}\%$, $FEF_{75-85}\%$, and $FEF_{200-1200}$. All of these have marked variability in normal subjects and very wide 95% confidence intervals which limits their clinical usefulness. The FVC maneuver should be performed a minimum of three times, but as many attempts as needed to reach reproducibility criteria. For valid results, the largest FVC and second-largest FVC should vary by no more than 5% or 100 ml, whichever is greater. The largest FEV_1

and second largest FEV$_1$ should meet the same criteria. Results should be recorded from the single best FEV1 and single best FVC.

Reference: pages 133, 134

Answer 8.3.   C - True; A, B, D - False

Flow volume curves have a characteristic appearance during forced exhalation. The initial one-third of the exhalation from TLC (from beginning to peak flow), is effort dependent. The subsequent two-thirds of expiratory flow is effort independent. The patterns of curve concavity correlate with the degree of airway obstruction. Restrictive lung disease results in preservation of the relationship between volume and flow but with smaller total values. See Figure 8.4, page 135, *Chest Medicine,* 3rd edition.

Reference: pages 134, 135

Answer 8.4.   B - True; A, C, D - False

The peak expiratory flow (PEF) is an effort dependent measure of the highest flow rate possible during a forced exhalation from TLC. PEF meters are portable and inexpensive, providing asthma patients with an objective home measurement of their disease activity. Bronchoprovocation tests usually involve inhalation of known amounts of either histamine or methacholine, though other agents may be used. A 20% decline in FEV$_1$ after exposure of 8.0 mmol or less of the agent used is indicative of a "positive" test. Smokers with existing obstructive ventilatory impairment commonly have a positive response to methacholine indicating a high incidence of airway hyperresponsiveness in this group.

Reference: pages 135, 136

Answer 8.5.   B, C

Total lung capacity (TLC) can be determined by either gas dilution techniques or body plethysmography. The gas dilution techniques (with closed-circuit helium dilution or multibreath nitrogen washout) require the patient to begin and end the test at the end of a normal expiration, in order to determine functional residual capacity (FRC). Both methods are sensitive to errors from leakage of gas, and also fail to measure the volume of gas in lung bullae. Plethysmographic volume measurements may differ from the results obtained by using gas dilution or washout methods. Plethysmography measures both communication and non-communicating compartments, while gas dilution techniques measure only communicating airways. As with gas dilution, accuracy of plethysmography is dependent on initiating the test at the end of a normal expiration.

Reference: pages 136–138

Answer 8.6.   B, C - True; A, D - False

Airway resistance (R$_{AW}$) is the driving pressure divided by the flow that results from the pressure differential, and must be measured during air flow. Flow rates less than 0.5 liter/sec do not reflect the dynamic compression of the airways, and should be used. The distensibility of the lungs is assessed by measuring lung compliance. Lung compliance is determined by measuring lung volumes with a spirometer, and the pressure changes for a given change in volume, as measured by airway pressure and pleural pressure (estimated by measuring esophageal pressure). Static lung compliance is the measured compliance at a specific volume. It increases with advancing age and emphysema, and decreases with alveolar filling diseases and pulmonary fibrosis. Total lung compliance includes both pulmonary and chest wall factors.

Reference: pages 138, 139

Answer 8.7.   **A, C, D**

The diffusion capacity of the lungs is a measure of the ability of gases to diffuse from the alveoli to the blood. Diffusion capacity for carbon monoxide (CO) is most commonly measured, as CO is not normally present in the blood or lungs, and is much more soluble in blood than in lung tissue. Resistance to diffusion of carbon monoxide (DLCO) from alveoli to blood is equally dependent on two major factors: the state of the alveolar-capillary membrane and the hemoglobin content in the pulmonary capillaries. Several methods are available to measure DLCO, with the single-breath method being the most commonly performed due to its simplicity; however, it may give errant results due to its sensitivity to ventilation-perfusion abnormalities. Measurements of DLCO are decreased when the surface area for gas exchange is reduced. Abnormalities in DLCO due to lung size can be assessed by correcting for alveolar volume (DLCO/VA). A correction factor for abnormal hemoglobin levels should also be used prior to assessing the presence or absence of diffusion abnormalities.

Reference: pages 141–143

Answer 8.8:   **B, C - True; A, D - False**

The best metabolic index of the work capacity in a given individual is the maximum oxygen consumption per unit time (VO_{2max}). Estimation of VO_2 from nomograms does not account for the contribution of anaerobic metabolism to VO_2, and this indirect estimate of the VO_2 tends to overestimate improvements in VO_2 on repeated testing. The cardiac output is the limiting factor for VO_{2max} in normal subjects, but is dependent primarily on an increased heart rate with stroke volume playing a proportionately smaller role.

Reference: pages 144–146

Answer 8.9.   **B, C, D**

Ventilatory capacity is usually the limiting factor of exercise capacity in patients with lung disease. Both normal individuals and those with lung disease are unable to maintain minute ventilation above 60% of MVV without developing dyspnea and muscle fatigue. Patients with lung disease have a reduced ventilatory reserve and increased ventilatory requirements, which is determined by CO_2 production, $PaCO_2$, and dead space ventilation fraction of each breath (VD/VT). Dead space ventilation normally decreases in normal subjects, but may remain unchanged in patients with COPD.

Reference: pages 147, 148

Answer 8.10.   **D**

Training improves exercise performance capacity primarily due to an increase in cardiac output. The cardiac output increases as a result of a maximum stroke volume due to improved cardiac function. Peripheral vascular resistance decreases, also improving cardiac output. Exercising muscle receives an increased distribution of the cardiac output facilitating an increase in oxidative capacity, mitochondrial enzymes, and promotion of the use of free fatty acids as fuel. In contrast, COPD patients do not increase mitochondrial activity with exercise, and their VO_{2max} usually does not increase by more than 10% during a training program.

Reference: pages 147–150

Evaluation and Management of Lung Disease

chapter 9

ASTHMA

QUESTIONS

Question 9.1. **Which of the following statements is true concerning asthma?**

A. Mortality from asthma has remained steady over the past twenty years for most industrialized countries, but is rising in the United States.
B. Morbidity and mortality are increasing in the U.S., with the increase most marked among men.
C. Mortality attributed to asthma has significantly increased since 1980 in the U.S.
D. Incidence of asthma is estimated to be approximately 8–12% of the United States population.
E. Mortality rates in the U.S. are rising more rapidly among Caucasians than black Americans.

Question 9.2. **A 24-year-old male college student presents to the emergency room with rapid onset of dyspnea and anxiety over the past hour. Examination shows an ill appearing man with a pulse rate of 106, BP 134/76, respiratory rate 28 and wheezing over both lung fields. Peak expiratory flow is 120L/m and chest x-ray reveals only hyperinflation, with low, flat diaphragms. Regarding this patient's disease:**

A. He should receive inhaled albuterol and oral theophylline, and be instructed to return to the emergency room if his symptoms persist.
B. He should receive albuterol and theophylline, plus a peak flow meter for home use, and be instructed to measure peak flow rate every two hours.
C. He should receive subcutaneous epinephrine, IV theophylline, and inhaled albuterol, and told to return to the emergency room if symptoms persist over three hours.
D. He should receive inhaled corticosteroids as part of his emergency room therapy.
E. Treatment should include intravenous corticosteroids and close observation until peak expiratory flow rate and symptoms improve.

Question 9.3. **A 41-year-old black woman presents to the emergency department with a history of seasonal rhinitis, episodic shortness of breath, and episodic wheezing for which she uses an albuterol inhaler. She does not smoke cigarettes. On exam, she is noted to have severely decreased air movement and cyanosis. Blood gases confirm profound hypoxia and the patient is endotracheally intubated and mechanically ventilated. Despite appropriate treatment with beta agonists, corticosteroids, and aminophylline, the patient expires three days after admission. At autopsy, pathologic findings would likely include all of the following EXCEPT:**

A. Infiltration with neutrophils and smooth muscle hypertrophy.
B. Thickened basement membranes and mucosal edema.
C. Epithelial desquamation

D. Mucus plugs containing epithelial cells and proteinaceous and cellular components of the inflammatory reaction.

Question 9.4.   **Major therapeutic actions of beta adrenergic agonists include all of the following EXCEPT:**

A. Bronchodilation
B. Facilitation of mucociliary clearance
C. Inhibition of acute mediator release from mast cells
D. Decrease in cellular inflammation

Question 9.5.   **While mowing lawns during spring break, a 19-year-old asthmatic college student (baseline PEFR 400 L/m) has an acute deterioration in respiratory status. Upon presentation to the emergency room, he appears to be in severe distress with a respiratory rate of 32, BP 136/80 (which falls to 122/76 with inspiration), and a pulse rate of 132 bpm. PEFR is 180 L/m. Wheezing is not appreciated on chest exam. Concerning the severity of this patient's disease, which of the following statements is true?**

A. The presence of an elevated heart rate, respiratory rate, and pulsus paradoxus is evidence of severe airflow obstruction.
B. Beta agonists alone are adequate to prevent the late asthmatic response that is expected to occur in 6–8 hours.
C. The lack of cyanosis is good evidence that the patient's gas exchange is adequate.
D. The absence of wheezing during an asthma attack indicates relatively mild bronchospasm, and suggests rapid recovery.

Question 9.6.   **A 53-year-old moderately obese black woman is referred for evaluation because of three hospitalizations in the preceding four months for asthma. She reports nighttime dyspepsia and severe wheezing with a cough productive of brownish sputum. Her medications include ketoprofen for rheumatoid arthritis and lisinopril for hypertension. Regarding this patient, which of the following statements is FALSE?**

A. Gastro-esophageal reflux disease (GERD) may be contributing to the patient's asthma symptoms.
B. Ketoprofen, but not lisinopril, is known to cause drug induced asthma.
C. A chest radiograph with parenchymal infiltrates coupled with high serum IgE levels and peripheral eosinophilia is good evidence that the patient has allergic bronchopulmonary aspergillosis (ABPA).
D. A 100% increase in serum IgE levels in a patient with ABPA warrants resumption of corticosteroid therapy.

Question 9.7.   **A 36-year-old Caucasian woman presents to your office with dyspnea and wheezing, which are more severe than during her usual mild asthmatic attacks. She receives albuterol 5 mg via nebulizer twice, 30 minutes apart. Her PEFR improves from 180 L/m to 320 L/m (her baseline), and she is discharged with a new prescription for albuterol MDI with a spacer device. The emergency room physician phones later that evening stating that the patient is in status asthmaticus. Concerning this patient's case and therapy, determine whether the following statements are TRUE or FALSE:**

A. The patient's decline in respiratory status is likely due to the "late asthmatic response" (LAR) which could have been blocked by a "long acting" beta agonist, such as salmeterol.

B. Chronic therapy with oral corticosteroids is the only proven effective means of blocking both the early and late asthmatic responses.
C. The biphasic decline in this patient's respiratory status could have been prevented by continuing albuterol nebulization therapy for a minimum of 6–8 hours.
D. The LAR can be blocked by either corticosteroids or nedocromil.

Question 9.8. **A family practitioner refers a 43-year-old man who is obese and complains of a non-productive cough with episodic shortness of breath. Chest film is normal, as is his spirogram. Regarding the initial evaluation of this patient, which of the following statements are TRUE or FALSE?**

A. Specific questions concerning nocturnal symptoms should be asked.
B. A bronchoprovocation test is useful to detect airway hyperactivity in cough-variant asthma.
C. Asthma "mimics," such as gastro-esophageal reflux and congestive heart failure, can cause similar presenting symptoms.
D. Bronchoscopy is likely to be beneficial in identifying this patient's problem.

Question 9.9. **A 22-year-old medical student is referred from the student health clinic with complaints of episodic dyspnea and wheezing over the past several weeks. He has a history of childhood asthma but has been asymptomatic for twelve years. He describes brief episodes of wheezing occurring about once every two weeks. Spirometry is normal. Which of the following statements are TRUE or FALSE?**

A. This patient is classified as having moderate asthma and should be started on an inhaled β-agonist as well as an anti-inflammatory drug such as an inhaled corticosteroid or cromolyn.
B. Sustained release oral theophylline is indicated for mild asthma, to prevent nocturnal symptoms.
C. Ipratropium bromide has been found to be as effective as inhaled β-adrenergic agents in the treatment of mild asthma.
D. Treatment with as-needed inhaled β-agonists alone is appropriate therapy at this time.

Question 9.10. **Concerning β-adrenergic agonists as used in the treatment of asthma, which of the following statements are TRUE or FALSE?**

A. The mechanism of action is through activation of adenyl cyclase, increasing intracellular c-AMP.
B. Oral delivery of β-adrenergic agents has a similar side effect profile to that of aerosol delivery.
C. Tachycardia due to "selective" β-2 agonists may be due to "crossover" with β-1 stimulation as well as a reflex response to peripheral vasodilatation.
D. Breath activated powder inhalers require more patient coordination than metered dose inhalers.

ANSWERS

Answer 9.1. **C**

Data from the National Center for Health Statistics from 1980–89 show that age-adjusted death rate for asthma increased from 1.3 per 100,000 population to 1.9 per 100,000 population. This reflects a worldwide increase in mortality rates among industrialized nations. This represents a 46% overall increase (54% for females and 23% for males) in the U.S. Also during this period, death rates for blacks was consistently higher than for whites, and the increase in death rate for black males is twice that for white males. Black and white females had similar rates of increase.

Reference: pages 163–165

Answer 9.2. **E**

This man has had rapid onset of severe bronchospasm, over a period of one hour. Wasserfallen has noted three patterns of asthma decompensation in terms of delay of symptom onset and endotracheal intubation. The acute asphyxia group was more common in men and had an onset to decompensation average of three hours. A proposed mechanism is bronchospasm causing extreme hypercapnia resulting in respiratory arrest. The group with gradual onset of symptoms had a delay in decompensation of 9.2 ± 7.7 days, and the "unstable asthmatics" with acute deterioration had a delay of 4.2 ± 3.6 days.

Reference: pages 165–166

Answer 9.3. **A**

At autopsy, pathologic findings of patients with asthma show evidence of airway inflammation as a fundamental part of acute asthma attacks. These findings include infiltration with eosinophils, smooth muscle hypertrophy, thickened basement membranes, mucosal edema, epithelial desquamation, and mucus plugs containing epithelial cells and proteinaceous and cellular components of the inflammatory response.

Reference: page 167

Answer 9.4. **D**

β-agonists have many beneficial effects upon patients with acute asthma exacerbations, including smooth muscle relaxation (bronchodilation), enhancement of mucus clearance, and inhibition of release of mediators from mast cells. They are the best bronchodilating agents known, however they do not decrease the inflammation of airways, and they do not affect the late asthmatic response (LAR).

Reference: page 176

Answer 9.5. **A**

Objective findings associated with severe airflow obstruction include PEFR <120 L/m, FEV_1 <1L, HR:130, RR>30, and pulsus paradoxus. None of these findings, alone or in combination, is specific for determining need for hospitalization, and sound clinical judgement remains a mainstay in addressing this issue.

Reference: pages 170–172

Answer 9.6. **B**

The workup of a patient presenting with recurrent episodes of bronchospasm should include the exclusion of a number of conditions. These include upper airway obstruction, gastro-esophageal reflux, allergic bronchopulmonary aspergillosis (ABPA), and drug induced bronchospasm. This patient's history is significant for the presence of gastro-esophageal reflux as well as possible drug induced symptoms. Non-steroidal anti-inflammatory agents (ketoprofen), ACE inhibitors (lisinopril), and β-blockers are known to induce cough and wheezing. ABPA is unlikely in this patient. The need for therapy in ABPA is based on clinical findings plus a marked increase in serum IgE levels.

Reference: pages 172–173

Answer 9.7.   **D - True; A, B, C - False**

The early asthmatic response occurs immediately, persists up to 3 to 4 hours, and can be prevented with inhaled β-adrenergic agonists. The late asthmatic response (LAR), occurs after several hours, and is not prevented by adrenergic agonists. The LAR can be prevented by either inhaled, oral, or parenteral corticosteroids, cromolyn, or nedocromil.

Reference: pages 183–189.

Answer 9.8.   **A, B, C - True; D - False**

This patient likely has asthma, although other possibilities such as gastro-esophageal reflux must be considered. Cough-variant asthma may be unmasked by bronchoprovocation tests or careful monitoring of variation in flow rates over time. Bronchoscopy is indicated if a flow-volume loop suggests upper airway obstruction, if the chest film reveals a pulmonary or mediastinal lesion, or if other symptoms such as hemoptysis are reported.

Reference: pages 170–172

Answer 9.9.   **D - True; A, B, C - False**

The patient is classified as having mild asthma, as he is having brief bi-weekly episodes of dyspnea. Therapy for mild asthma is as-needed β-agonists. Moderate asthma is more frequent in occurrence and accompanied by a PEFR or FEV_1 below 80% of baseline with 20 to 30% variation. Moderate asthma therapy should include β-agonists and inhaled corticosteroids or cromolyn. Theophylline may be added for nocturnal symptoms.

Reference: pages 175–184

Answer 9.10.   **A, C - True; B, D - False**

Oral β-adrenergic agonists are subject to patient-to-patient variability in absorption and first pass hepatic metabolism. Since they are absorbed systemically, they have more side effects than inhaled agents. Aerosol delivery of β-agonists is associated with a more rapid onset of action and has significantly fewer side effects than oral agents. Side effects with inhaled β-agonists are mild and are usually limited to tachycardia (mainly reflex due to vasodilation) and muscle tremor (a β-2 effect). These side effects decrease with continued use. These agents are thought to act primarily by activation of cellular adenyl cyclase, causing an increase in cyclic-AMP, which results in smooth muscle relaxation and stabilization of cell membranes. Breath activated powder inhalers require less patient coordination than metered dose inhalers.

Reference: pages 176–178

[handwritten margin note: peripheral vasodilation + reflex tachy.]

chapter 10

Chronic Obstructive Lung Diseases:

Emphysema, Chronic Bronchitis, Bronchiectasis,

and Cystic Fibrosis

QUESTIONS

Question 10.1. **Which of the following is/are cardinal pathologic features of chronic bronchitis?**

A. Enlargement of the mucus-secreting elements in the airways.
B. An increase in the fraction of mucous versus serous glands.
C. Narrowing and inflammation of small airways (2-mm diameter or smaller).
D. Development of bronchoscopically visible diverticula in the airways.

Question 10.2. **Which of the following statements is/are correct regarding the definition of emphysema?**

A. The definition specifies pathologic rather than clinical features.
B. Consists of air space enlargement beyond the terminal bronchiole and destruction of the alveolar wall.
C. Air space enlargement is permanent.
D. Fibrosis and repair are features of emphysema.

Question 10.3. **Which of the following statements is/are correct concerning the epidemiology of COPD?**

A. In 1991, COPD became the fourth leading cause of death in the United States.
B. COPD is the largest component of lung-related health care costs.
C. Trends over the past two decades have shown an increase in the prevalence of COPD and an increase in age-adjusted mortality.
D. Emphysema is the most prevalent form of COPD.

Question 10.4. **Which of the following statements is/are correct regarding the influenza vaccine?**

A. Current recommendations call for administration of the vaccine yearly to patients with COPD.
B. The vaccine will often cause symptoms of fever, malaise, and myalgias.
C. The vaccine can be administered concurrently with the pneumococcal vaccine.
D. The vaccine consists of a live attenuated egg-grown virus, usually a combination of A and B strains.

Question 10.5. **Which of the following statements is/are correct regarding the use of theophylline in patients with COPD?**

A. Patients on theophylline may show an improvement in functional status without any improvement in air flow.
B. Theophylline may be beneficial in improving the function of respiratory muscles.
C. A potential side effect of theophylline is the occurrence of supraventricular tachycardias.
D. Theophylline is the initial treatment of choice in patients with acute exacerbations of COPD.

Question 10.6. Which of the following statements is/are correct regarding the use of corticosteroids in patients with COPD?

A. Corticosteroids have been shown to decrease recovery time in patients with acute exacerbations of COPD.
B. Corticosteroids have been shown to be beneficial in 10–50% of patients with stable COPD.
C. Corticosteroid trials should be considered when a patient remains functionally impaired after conventional therapy.
D. A single dose of intravenous methylprednisolone (100 mg) has been shown to be as beneficial as a 3-day course in acute exacerbations of chronic bronchitis.

Question 10.7. Which of the following statements is/are correct concerning the use of supplemental oxygen in patients with COPD?

A. Oxygen administration improves survival in patients with stable, hypoxemic COPD.
B. Continuous oxygen therapy has been shown to decrease pulmonary vascular resistance in patients with stable, hypoxemic COPD.
C. Continuous oxygen therapy has been shown to decrease the level of polycythemia in patients with stable, hypoxemic COPD
D. Oxygen administration improves survival in patients with acute hypoxemic exacerbations of COPD.

Question 10.8. Demonstrated short-term benefits of pulmonary rehabilitation in patients with COPD include which of the following?

A. Improved endurance of specific muscle groups
B. Improved functional status
C. Improved exercise capacity
D. Improved strength of specific muscle groups

Question 10.9. Augmentation therapy with purified α_1-antitrypsin for patients with α_1-antitrypsin deficiency is suggested for patients meeting which of the following criteria?

A. Serum α_1-antitrypsin level less than 11 µM.
B. Expected patient compliance.
C. Abnormal lung function consistent with emphysema.
D. Age above 18 years unless obstructive lung disease is present earlier.

Question 10.10. Treatment of cystic fibrosis consists of which of the following regimens?

A. Gene therapy
B. Correction of abnormal salt transport
C. Decreasing viscosity of airway mucus
D. Modulation of airway inflammation

Question 10.11. **Cigarette smoking promotes alveolar breakdown in emphysema by all of the following mechanisms EXCEPT:**

A. Recruiting elastase-rich neutrophils to alveoli
B. Antigenic stimulation of CD4 lymphocytes
C. Inactivating α_1-antitrypsin
D. Opposing elastin resynthesis

Question 10.12. **One of the cardinal manifestations of chronic bronchitis is the colonization of airways by bacteria. Which of the following is NOT a commonly found organism in the airways of chronic bronchitis patients?**

A. *Streptococcus pneumoniae*
B. *Haemophilus influenzae*
C. *Staphylococcus aureus*
D. *Moraxella catarrhalis*

Question 10.13. **Which of the following statements is correct concerning the use of amantadine for influenza A prophylaxis?**

A. In influenza A outbreaks, amantadine can provide effective chemoprophylaxis in nearly 100% of cases.
B. Amantadine may reduce the duration of influenza A-related symptoms if administered up to 72–96 hours after the onset of viral disease.
C. The usual adult dose is 200 mg once daily; since it is metabolized by the liver, no adjustments are needed for patients with impaired renal function.
D. Amantadine may be used as an adjunct to late immunization in patients at high risk for influenza A infection.

Question 10.14. **The use of anticholinergic bronchodilators would be preferred over sympathomimetic agents in all of the following clinical conditions EXCEPT:**

A. Bronchospasm precipitated by β-blockers
B. Air flow obstruction in stable COPD
C. Acute bronchospasm in late onset adult asthma
D. Bronchospasm precipitated by psychogenic causes

Question 10.15. **Which of the following statements concerning α_1-antitrypsin deficiency is INCORRECT?**

A. α_1-antitrypsin deficiency accounts for 2–5% of all cases of emphysema.
B. α_1-antitrypsin is a glycoprotein synthesized in the liver which serves as the major inactivator of neutrophil-derived elastase.
C. α_1-antitrypsin variants differ in protein structure or in gene expression, with all variants causing a similar decrease in serum levels of α_1-antitrypsin.
D. The disorder is codominantly inherited, and over 75 different alleles have been identified.

Question 10.16. **Persons with which of the following α_1-antitrypsin phenotypes would be at highest risk for developing emphysema?**

A. PiZZ
B. Pi Null Null
C. PiMZ
D. PiMS

Question 10.17. Which of the following conditions has NOT been recognized as being associated with development of bronchiectasis?

A. Panhypogammaglobulinemia
B. Kartagener's syndrome
C. Cystic fibrosis
D. Loeffler's syndrome

Question 10.18. Which of the following statements is correct with regards to pulmonary manifestations of cystic fibrosis?

A. The presence of mucoid *Pseudomonas* in the sputum is diagnostic of cystic fibrosis.
B. The chest radiograph is normal in only about 2% of adults with cystic fibrosis.
C. Bronchiectatic changes tend to occur first in the left upper lobe.
D. Pulmonary function tests usually reveal a restrictive impairment.

Question 10.19. Which of the following bacterial species is NOT a predominant cause of lung infections in patients with cystic fibrosis?

A. *Pseudomonas aeruginosa*
B. *Haemophilus influenzae*
C. *Pseudomonas cepacia*
D. *Moraxella catarrhalis*

Question 10.20. Match the anatomic category of emphysema to the clinical findings:

1. May be most apparent in the bases of the lungs on chest radiograph.
2. May present as spontaneous pneumothorax.
3. Classically associated with α_1-antitrypsin deficiency.
4. Results from long-term cigarette smoking.
5. Emphysema is extensive with minimal air flow obstruction.
6. Most commonly seen in upper lung zones on chest radiograph.

A. Centriacinar
B. Panacinar
C. Distal acinar

Question 10.21. Match the lettered statements with the numbered comments below:

1. Decreased FEV_1/FVC ratio
2. Normal diffusion capacity
3. Increased residual volume
4. Cor pulmonale
5. Decreased total lung capacity

A. Present in chronic bronchitis
B. Present in emphysema
C. Present in both chronic bronchitis and emphysema
D. Present in neither chronic bronchitis nor emphysema

Question 10.22. Match the lettered type of bronchodilator agent to the numbered characteristic below:

1. Peak of bronchodilation within 5 minutes
2. Peak of bronchodilation after about 30 minutes
3. Bronchodilation occurs in larger and more central airways

4. Bronchodilation occurs in more peripheral airways
5. Best given by inhalation to avoid systemic effects

A. Sympathomimetic bronchodilators
B. Anticholinergic bronchodilators
C. Both sympathomimetic and anticholinergic bronchodilators

Question 10.23. **TRUE/FALSE - The following findings may be seen on the chest radiographs of patients with emphysema:**

A. Flattened diaphragm
B. Irregular radiolucency of lung fields
C. Decrease in peripheral vasculature
D. Increased retrosternal space
E. Indentation ("scalloping") of portions of the diaphragm
F. "Deep sulcus sign" on the supine film

Question 10.24. **TRUE/FALSE - The following statements are True or False regarding the pneumococcal vaccine:**

A. Pneumococcal vaccine is recommended for patients with chronic illness and otherwise healthy adults over 65 years of age.
B. Individuals who received the original 14-valent vaccine should be revaccinated with the newer 23-valent vaccine.
C. Mild local reactions occur in about one-half of patients receiving the vaccine; anaphylactoid reactions are rare.
D. COPD patients who are colonized with *Streptococcus pneumoniae* will often have pre-vaccination serum antibody titers above protective thresholds.

Question 10.25. **TRUE/FALSE - Determine whether the following statements are TRUE or FALSE concerning antibiotic therapy in patients with acute exacerbations of COPD:**

A. The use of antibiotics has been shown to improve rate of resolution and decrease the incidence of deterioration.
B. Gram stain and culture are not useful in exacerbations due to the presence of colonized bacteria in COPD patients, and have no effect on the choice of antibiotics.
C. The greatest benefit of antibiotics is seen in patients with increases in dyspnea, sputum production, and purulence.

Question 10.26. **TRUE/FALSE - Determine if the following statements are TRUE or FALSE regarding the clinical aspects of α_1-antitrypsin deficiency:**

A. Chest radiographs typically show bullous disease in the apices.
B. Pulmonary function tests frequently reveal obstruction of air flow and a decrease in diffusion capacity.
C. PiZZ α_1-antitrypsin disease is strongly associated with concomitant liver disease.
D. Patients with α_1-antitrypsin deficiency who have never smoked may develop symptoms later than smokers.

Question 10.27. **TRUE/FALSE - Determine whether the following statements are TRUE or FALSE regarding cystic fibrosis:**

A. Cystic fibrosis is the most common fatal inherited disease in Caucasians.
B. The main pathophysiologic abnormality is a defect in electrolyte transport causing a decrease in sodium absorption from the airway lumen.
C. The discovery of the cystic fibrosis gene allows for detection in 95% of carriers.

D. Patients with cystic fibrosis usually present in early childhood or adolescence, with diagnosis made in all patients before age 20.

ANSWERS

Answer 10.1. **All are correct**

Enlargement of the mucus-secreting elements consists of an increase in both the number of glands and in their size (hypertrophy), characterized by dilation of the ducts and enlargement of the secretory cells. Narrowing and inflammation of small airways and a deficit of small airways with specific size ranges are also pathologic features in chronic bronchitis. Bronchoscopically visible diverticula in the walls of airways are another pathologic hallmark; these are believed to represent dilated openings of mucous glands; they range in size from 0.2–1.2 mm in diameter.

[handwritten: terminal bronchiole]

Reference: page 202

Answer 10.2. **A, B, C**

All available definitions of emphysema specify pathologic rather than clinical features as diagnostic criteria. Key pathologic features of emphysema include air space enlargement beyond the terminal bronchiole and destruction of the alveolar wall. Refinements of the previous ATS definition have included specifying that air space enlargements are permanent and that fibrosis is not a feature of true emphysema.

Reference: page 202

Answer 10.3. **A, C**

In 1991, chronic obstructive pulmonary disease (including asthma, bronchiectasis, and hypersensitivity pneumonitis) became the fourth leading cause of death of Americans. Trends over the past two decades suggest a 60.4% increase in the prevalence of COPD through 1987; mortality trends suggest recent increases in age-related mortality from COPD, which has risen by 37.7% from 1979 to 1991. The total 1986 cost of all lung diseases collectively was over $40 billion, with COPD (23.5%) second only to lung cancer (26.4%) as the largest component. Data from the National Health Interview Survey (NHIS) of 1991 suggest that chronic bronchitis is the most prevalent type of COPD (12.5 million Americans), followed by emphysema (1.6 million Americans).

Reference: pages 202–203

Answer 10.4. **A, C**

Because influenza infection poses an increased risk of hospitalization and death in patients with COPD, current recommendations call for administering the influenza vaccine yearly to these patients. The vaccine consists of an inactivated egg-grown virus, almost always a trivalent combination of two A virus strains and one B virus strain. The influenza vaccine can be administered concurrently with the pneumococcal vaccine (though at a different site) and infrequently causes self-limited constitutional symptoms of fever, malaise, and myalgias.

Reference: page 216

Answer 10.5. **A, B, C**

Support for using theophylline in patients with stable COPD comes from studies showing that theophylline can enhance patients' functional status and improve dyspnea even in the absence of bronchodilation. Further studies suggest that the beneficial effects of theophylline on dyspnea and functional status in stable COPD correlate most closely with improvements in respiratory muscle function. A distinctive potential complication of theophylline in COPD is the development of multifocal atrial tachycardia, a rapid but irregular supraventricular tachycardia characterized by at least three separate P wave morphologies. Originally believed to reflect the sequelae of underlying lung disease, its occurrence as a manifestation of theophylline toxicity has more recently been suggested. Recent data suggest that theophylline confers at best only a marginal benefit in treating patients with acute exacerbations of COPD.

Reference: pages 220–221

Answer 10.6.   **A, B, C**

The use of corticosteroids, both inhaled and systemic, continues to be a source of much debate. Overall, it appears that corticosteroids are beneficial in 10–56% of patients with stable COPD, and that individual patients may show varying degrees of improvement. Corticosteroid trials should be considered when stable COPD patients remain functionally impaired despite optimal conventional therapy (e.g., inhaled β-2 adrenergic agonists and anticholinergics, theophylline, pulmonary rehabilitation). As with acute exacerbations of asthma, corticosteroids have been shown to be effective in accelerating recovery from acute exacerbations of COPD. Recent studies suggest that unlike a 3-day course of intravenous methylprednisolone, a single 100-mg dose in the emergency room does not accelerate improvement during an acute exacerbation of chronic bronchitis.

Reference: pages 221–222

Answer 10.7.   **All are correct**

Supplemental oxygen therapy is a key aspect of treating patients with hypoxic COPD, because oxygen has shown to benefit patients with acute hypoxemic exacerbations of COPD, as well as patients with chronic, stable COPD. Results from two important studies regarding oxygen administration therapy, the British Medical Research Council (MRC) study and the American Nocturnal Oxygen Therapy Trial (NOTT), have shown that oxygen therapy improves survival in patients with stable, hypoxemic COPD. Other benefits of oxygen therapy in the American trial included significantly decreased pulmonary vascular resistance and a greater amelioration of polycythemia in patients treated with continuous oxygen therapy.

Reference: page 223

Answer 10.8.   **All are correct**

A pulmonary rehabilitation program can be a useful adjunct to medical therapy for patients with stable COPD. Demonstrated short-term benefits of pulmonary rehabilitation include improved strength and/or endurance of the specific muscle groups trained, improved exercise capacity, and improved functional status.

Reference: page 225

Answer 10.9.   **All are correct**

According to the current treatment guidelines of the American Thoracic Society, augmentation therapy is suggested for patients with α_1-antitrypsin deficiency who satisfy all the criteria listed. Candidates must be homozygous for the deficiency, and must have evidence of emphysema, but must not be end stage. Replacement therapy will not improve lung function; the aim is only to prevent further damage.

Reference: page 231

Answer 10.10.   **All are correct**

In April 1993, the National Heart, Lung, and Blood Institute announced the start of the first gene therapy trials for treating cystic fibrosis. The gene therapy technique under study involves the instillation into the airway of an adenovirus containing the normal human gene for CFTR, with the goal of transfecting the host CF patient's respiratory epithelial cells. Amiloride can block the uptake of sodium from the airway by respiratory epithelium, resulting in an increased mucus water content and improved clearance of secretions. The presence of polymerized DNA from degenerating leukocytes significantly increases the viscosity of airway secretions. The use of aerosolized recombinant DNASE has been shown to be well tolerated and to result in significant improvement in lung function. A recent study has shown that aerosolized leukoprotease inhibitor results in a significant decrease in interleukin-8, neutrophil elastase levels, and neutrophil numbers on the respiratory epithelial lining fluid of cystic fibrosis patients, resulting in decreased damage to epithelial cells and less airway inflammation.

Reference: page 236

Answer 10.11.   **B**

As a major risk factor for emphysema, cigarette smoking promotes alveolar breakdown in several ways: *(a)* by recruiting elastase-rich neutrophils to alveoli; *(b)* by inactivating α_1-antitrypsin, both directly by oxidant products of combustion and indirectly through oxidant products of neutrophils; and *(c)* by opposing elastin resynthesis, a result of diminished activity of the enzyme (lysyl oxidase) responsible for cross-linking newly synthesized elastin fibrils. CD4 lymphocyte stimulation has not been implicated as a mechanism of injury in emphysema caused by cigarette smoke.

Reference: pages 208–209

Answer 10.12.   **C**

Colonization of normally sterile airways occurs in patients with chronic bronchitis. During exacerbations, patients will often present with an increase in production of purulent sputum. Sputum examination most frequently shows *Haemophilus influenzae, Streptococcus pneumoniae,* or *Moraxella catarrhalis,* all of which are common organisms of the normal upper respiratory tract.

Reference: pages 204, 222

Answer 10.13.   **D**

In the event of an influenza A outbreak, amantadine can provide chemoprophylaxis with 70–90% efficacy. Amantadine may also reduce the duration of influenza A-related constitutional symptoms if administered within 48 hours of the onset of viral disease. The usual adult dose is 200 mg once daily, but the dose is reduced to 100 mg once daily for patients aged 65 or above or for patients with impaired renal function. Amantadine is best used as an adjunct to late immunization in patients at high risk for influenza A infection, so treatment should persist only until an antibody response is expected (usually within 2 weeks of vaccination).

Reference: pages 216–217

Answer 10.14. **C**

Recent evidence recommends anticholinergic bronchodilators over sympathomimetic agents in several clinical settings: bronchospasm precipitated by β-blockers, air flow obstruction in stable COPD, and bronchospasm precipitated by psychogenic causes. Some studies also suggest the superiority of anticholinergic bronchodilators over sympathomimetic agents in acute exacerbations of COPD and in severe COPD. Sympathomimetic agents remain the bronchodilator of choice in acute asthma.

Reference: page 218

Answer 10.15. **C**

α_1-antitrypsin deficiency is an inherited disorder that predisposes to emphysema and accounts for 2–5% of all cases of emphysema. The disorder is codominantly inherited, with over 75 different alleles having been identified as of this publication. α_1-antitrypsin is a 52,000-dalton (394-amino acid) glycoprotein that is synthesized in the liver and that serves as the major inactivator of neutrophil-derived elastase. α_1-antitrypsin variants differ in protein structure or gene expression, with some variants preserving antiprotease activity and others impairing either synthesis or antiprotease activity.

Reference: page 229

Answer 10.16. **B**

Neither PiMZ nor PiMS has been clearly implicated as predisposing to emphysema. The most common phenotype with low levels and elevated risk is PiZZ; however, those individuals with Pi Null Null phenotype (in whom no α_1-antitrypsin is synthesized in the liver) are considered to be at even higher risk than PiZZ individuals.

Reference: page 229

Answer 10.17. **D**

Bronchiectasis is best classified according to the underlying cause or predisposing factor. Bronchiectasis is not a discrete entity, but rather represents the possible result of several different diseases or insults. With the decrease in pyogenic infections of the lungs, bronchiectasis is now more commonly due to abnormal host defenses such as is seen with cystic fibrosis, immunoglobulin deficiency states, and dyskinetic cilia syndromes. Loeffler's syndrome has not been associated with development of bronchiectasis.

Reference: pages 231–233

Answer 10.18. **B**

As cystic fibrosis progresses, mucoid strains of *Pseudomonas aeruginosa* often appear in the sputum. Such a finding is an important clue to the underlying diagnosis, but it is not entirely specific because mucoid *Pseudomonas* is also found in patients with bronchiectasis not caused by cystic fibrosis. The chest radiograph is normal in only about 2% of adults with cystic fibrosis. Bronchiectatic changes tend to occur first in the right upper lobe, followed by the left upper lobe and the right middle lobe. Pulmonary function tests almost always reveal an obstructive impairment; with scarring and fibrosis, restriction of lung volumes may occur at a later stage.

Reference: page 234

Answer 10.19. **D**

Four bacterial species predominate as causes of lung infection in cystic fibrosis patients: *Staphylococcus aureus*, *Haemophilus influenzae*, *Pseudomonas aeruginosa*, and *Pseudomonas cepacia*. Nontuberculous mycobacteria and viral infections have also been implicated in exacerbations of cystic fibrosis.

Reference: Page 236

Answer 10.20. **1-B; 2-C; 3-B; 4-A; 5-C; 6-A**

Centriacinar emphysema occurs with enlargement of the proximal portion of the acinus, the respiratory bronchiole. Centriacinar emphysema usually results from long-term cigarette smoking and begins in the upper lung zones on the chest radiograph. In contrast, panacinar emphysema involves the whole acinus, is classically associated with α_1-antitrypsin deficiency, and may be more apparent in the bases of the lung on the chest radiograph. Distal acinar emphysema involves the alveolar ducts and sacs farther out in the acinus. To the extent that these more distal acinar elements abut the pleura, distal acinar emphysema may present as a pneumothorax, as in the spontaneous pneumothorax that can occur in young patients. Also, because air-conducting elements of the airways are spared in the distal acinar form, emphysema can be extensive with little accompanying air flow obstruction.

Reference: page 202

Answer 10.21. **1-C; 2-A; 3-B; 4-C; 5-D**

Air flow is normally decreased in both emphysema and chronic bronchitis patients, with decreases seen in both the FEV_1 and the FEV_1/FVC ratio. Diffusion capacity is normal in chronic bronchitics, but decreased in emphysema patients due to alveolar damage. Increased residual volume is frequently seen in emphysema patients due to air trapping. Cor pulmonale, although more common in chronic bronchitis patients, does occur in emphysema patients, although it is usually later in the disease process. A decrease in total lung capacity is seen in neither instance; chronic bronchitis patients usually have normal lung volumes, whereas emphysema patients have increased lung volumes.

Reference: pages 209–210

Answer 10.22. **1-A; 2-B; 3-B; 4-A; 5-C**

The use of combination therapy with anticholinergic bronchodilators and sympathomimetic agents can be justified based on the different pharmacologic properties of each drug. Specifically, sympathomimetics tend to show an earlier onset of bronchodilation with a shorter duration, while anticholinergic agents exert a more delayed but prolonged effect. Large and central airways appear to be preferentially innervated by cholinergic fibers so that bronchodilation from anticholinergic drugs occurs centrally, in contrast to the effects of sympathomimetic agents, which are believed to act in more peripheral airways. Both types of agents are best administered by inhalation in order to provide maximum local effect with few systemic side effects.

Reference: pages 217–219.

Answer 10.23. **A, B, C, D, E -True; F - False**

The features of emphysema as noted on chest radiographs are divided into features of hyperinflation (e.g., depression and flattening of diaphragms, blunting of the costophrenic angles, increased length of the lung, increased size of the retrosternal air space) and features of vascular attenuation and hyperlucency (e.g., loss of lung parenchyma, bullous changes, and disappearance of vascular markings, especially in the lung periphery). The effects of large bullae on the film include rounded lucencies in the apex and base, and localized indentation of the diaphragm ("scalloping"). The "deep sulcus sign" on the supine chest film is evidence for a pneumothorax.

Reference: pages 212–213

Answer 10.24. **A, C, D - True; B - False**

The available pneumococcal vaccine is a 23-valent preparation that contains capsular antigens from pneumococcal serotypes that are responsible for 87% of bacteremic pneumococcal infections. Because of the increased risk for contracting pneumococcal infection and the increased mortality risk from infection in debilitated patients, pneumococcal vaccine has been recommended for adults with chronic illnesses (e.g., chronic pulmonary disease, cardiovascular disease, splenic dysfunction, Hodgkin's disease, myeloma, renal failure, and immunosuppression), as well as otherwise healthy adults aged 65 years and older. Individuals who received the earlier, 14-valent vaccine need not be revaccinated routinely with the 23-valent vaccine, but the Immunization Practices Advisory Committee recommends revaccination every 6 years after the first dose for individuals considered to be at high risk for rapid decline in antibody levels (e.g., chronic renal failure, nephrotic syndrome, or transplanted organs) or for potentially fatal pneumococcal infections (e.g., asplenic patients). Mild local reactions occur in roughly one-half of vaccine recipients; severe reactions and anaphylactoid reactions have been rarely described. Notably, COPD patients who are frequently colonized with streptococcal species will have pre-vaccination serum antibody titers to pneumococcal antigens that exceed protective thresholds, so the incremental value of vaccinating COPD patients may be small.

Reference: page 217

Answer 10.25. **A, C - True; B - False**

A study by Anthonisen and coworkers showed that successful resolution of acute exacerbations of COPD was 1.24 more likely in antibiotic recipients than in placebo recipients, and clinical deterioration beyond 72 hours after treatment was almost 2 times less likely in patients receiving antibiotics. The benefits of antibiotic therapy were greatest in patients who experienced the symptom triad of increased dyspnea, increased sputum volume, and increased purulence. Although Gram stain and cultures of sputum have not been deemed helpful in the initial management of acute exacerbations of COPD, the presence of *Moraxella catarrhalis* may affect antibiotic choice. Because 75% of *Moraxella catarrhalis* produce β-lactamase, identifying this organism on a Gram stain or culture should alter the initial choice of antibiotic.

Reference: pages 222–223

Answer 10.26. **B, C, D - True; A - False**

The most common clinical feature of affected individuals with αa_1-antitrypsin deficiency is emphysema of unusually early onset, commonly with chest x-ray evidence of basal bullae, unlike the usual apical location of bullae in smoking-related centriacinar emphysema. Although symptoms may begin in even young nonsmoking PiZZ individuals, current evidence suggests that those who have never smoked may develop symptoms somewhat later than smokers, with a mean delay in onset of 13 years. Pulmonary function tests show the expected pattern of air flow obstruction with severe declines in FEV_1 and relative preservation of forced vital capacity (FVC). Besides emphysema, PiZZ α_1-antitrypsin deficiency has been associated with a variety of other diseases. The strongest association is with liver disease, particularly neonatal hepatitis, cirrhosis, and hepatoma.

Reference: page 230

Answer 10.27. **A, C - True; B, D - False**

Cystic fibrosis is the most common fatal inherited disease in Caucasians. The main pathophysiologic abnormality is a defect in electrolyte transport. Decreased secretion of chloride into the airway lumen and increased sodium reabsorption from the airway lumen lead to a decrease in water content and increased viscosity of airway secretions. The discovery of the cystic fibrosis gene and the ability to detect the common "cystic fibrosis transmembrane conductance regulator" (CFTR) mutations now allow the routine screening of 33 mutations and the detection of 95% of carriers. Although cystic fibrosis is typically diagnosed in infancy or early childhood, a recent review found that 5% were diagnosed between 16 and 30 years of age. Less commonly, the diagnosis is made as late as 35 years of age.

Reference: page 234

chapter 11

Sleep-Related Breathing Disorders

QUESTIONS

Question 11.1. **Which of the following statements is/are correct concerning the effect of sleep on ventilation?**

A. Respiratory drive in non-REM sleep is reduced due solely to the loss of the stimulatory effect of wakefulness.
B. Intercostal and accessory respiratory muscle activity are reduced during REM sleep.
C. Human studies during non-REM sleep have shown an increase in tidal volume to help compensate for the lack of stimulation to breathe in order to maintain normal minute ventilation.
D. Stage REM is usually the stage of sleep most often associated with severe oxygen desaturation.

Question 11.2. **Which of the following conditions is NOT included in the tetrad of symptoms usually associated with narcolepsy?**

A. Sleep attacks
B. Hypnagogic hallucinations
C. Morning headaches
D. Sleep paralysis

Question 11.3. **Which of the following statements is/are correct concerning narcolepsy?**

A. Narcolepsy usually manifests initially in adolescence or early adulthood.
B. The hallmark of narcolepsy on a polysomnogram is the presence of sleep-onset stage REM.
C. Narcolepsy has been shown to have a genetic predisposition.
D. Treatment of narcolepsy involves the avoidance of stimulatory drugs and the use of serotonin-uptake inhibitors (e.g., Prozac, Zoloft).

Question 11.4. **Which of the following statements is/are correct concerning periodic limb movement (PLM) disorder?**

A. Ten percent of patients presenting to sleep centers with insomnia are found to have PLM as the major cause of their sleepiness.
B. Patients with excessive daytime sleepiness due to PLM usually complain of frequent leg movements associated with arousal from sleep.
C. Initial treatment of PLM is usually with tricyclic antidepressant drugs (protriptyline, imipramine).
D. The diagnosis of PLM requires EMG monitoring of both legs.

Question 11.5. **Conditions known to predispose patients to sleep apnea include all of the following EXCEPT:**

A. Male sex
B. Hypertension
C. Hypothyroidism
D. Alcohol use
E. Increasing age

Question 11.6. **Which of the following findings is/are normally seen on a polysomnogram of a patient with obstructive sleep apnea (OSA) syndrome?**

A. Paradoxical movements of the chest and abdomen.
B. Tachycardia during the apneic period and bradycardia during the postapnea arousal.
C. Arousal and movement coinciding with resumption of air flow after apnea.
D. A decrease in systemic blood pressure with apneic episodes.

Question 11.7. **The severity of desaturation seen in patients with OSA has been shown to correlate with which of the following factor(s)?**

A. Lower baseline PO_2
B. Smaller expiratory reserve volume
C. Higher apnea index
D. Greater percentage of sleep time spent in apnea

Question 11.8. **Which of the following statements is/are correct regarding the pathophysiology of upper airway obstruction in patients with obstructive sleep apnea (OSA)?**

A. The upper airway of OSA patients is abnormal during sleep, but normal airway patency is restored during wakefulness.
B. Patients with OSA usually have smaller than normal upper airways.
C. Fluctuations in neural drive to upper airway musculature as well as muscles of respiration are seen in patients with OSA.
D. The stimulus for arousal from apneic episodes during sleep in patients with OSA is regulated by the degree of oxygen desaturation and hypercapnia.

Question 11.9. **Which of the following statements is INCORRECT concerning daytime sleepiness in OSA?**

A. Sleep fragmentation is probably the most important factor causing excessive daytime somnolence.
B. Cognitive impairment is more severe in patients who have more severe arterial oxygen desaturation.
C. Pulse oximetry measurements are adequate to determine the severity of sleep disorder.
D. Treatment of sleep apnea via nasal CPAP will often result in a rapid improvement in daytime somnolence.

Question 11.10. **Which of the following statements is/are correct regarding nocturnal oxygen therapy as treatment for obstructive sleep apnea?**

A. Oxygenation improves with the use of nocturnal oxygen.
B. The frequency of apneic events decreases with nocturnal oxygen.
C. Improvements in morbidity are seen with the use of nocturnal oxygen.
D. The occurrence of cardiac arrhythmias may decrease with use of nocturnal oxygen.

Question 11.11.　Which of the following statements is/are correct regarding the use of nasal continuous positive airway pressure (CPAP) in patients with sleep apnea syndromes?

A. The most common problem associated with nasal CPAP is patient compliance.
B. Nasal CPAP has been shown to increase sleep latency on MSLT testing.
C. Nasal CPAP has been shown to decrease mortality in patients with OSA.
D. Nasal CPAP may be useful in improving daytime hypercapnia in patients with obesity hypoventilation syndrome.

Question 11.12.　Which of the following condition(s) lead to instability of ventilatory control in patients with central sleep apnea (CSA) associated with periodic breathing?

A. Low ventilatory response to hypoxia
B. Awake hypocapnia
C. Delayed neural feedback
D. Low oxygen stores

Question 11.13.　The following statements are TRUE/FALSE regarding hypercapnic central sleep apnea?

A. Patients with hypercapnic CSA usually present with respiratory failure and/or cor pulmonale.
B. Morning headaches and daytime hypersomnolence are uncommon.
C. The degree of oxygen desaturation is less severe than that seen in OSA.
D. The combination of supplemental oxygen and respiratory stimulants is the treatment of choice.

Question 11.14.　Which of the following statements is/are correct concerning the pathophysiologic mechanisms of nocturnal asthma?

A. The worst pulmonary function usually occurs around 4:00 AM.
B. An increase in circulating epinephrine is seen during normal sleep.
C. Patients with nocturnal asthma may have an increased infiltration of eosinophils during sleep.
D. Theophylline is more effective than inhaled β-agonists in preventing nocturnal asthma.

Question 11.15.　Which of the following statements is/are correct regarding the effects of sleep on patients with COPD?

A. Patients with COPD who exhibit CO_2 retention or resting hypoxia are more likely to exhibit severe desaturation during sleep.
B. Desaturation during stage REM is associated with reduced tidal volume and unchanged respiratory rate.
C. Nocturnal oxygen therapy decreases mortality in COPD patients with desaturations confined to stage REM sleep.
D. Patients with both COPD and OSA have more severe cardiopulmonary sequelae than those with equivalent amounts of sleep apnea.

ANSWERS

Answer 11.1.　**B, D**

Respiratory drive is reduced during non-REM sleep due to loss of the stimulatory effect of wakefulness and a decrease in chemosensitivity. Studies in humans during non-REM sleep have shown a reduction in minute ventilation associated with a decrease in tidal volume and either a decrease in respiratory rate or an increase not large enough to compensate for the fall in tidal volume. Intercostal and accessory muscle activity are reduced and functional residual capacity may also decrease during REM sleep. Stage REM is usually the stage of sleep associated with the most severe oxygen desaturation in patients with sleep-related respiratory disorders.

Reference: page 251

Answer 11.2. **C**

Narcolepsy is a syndrome associated with the tetrad of sleep attacks, cataplexy, hypnagogic hallucinations, and sleep paralysis. Although morning headaches may occur in some patients, they are not as common and are generally associated with the obstructive sleep apneas.

Reference: page 254

Answer 11.3. **A, B, C**

The attacks of sleepiness associated with narcolepsy usually begin in adolescence or early adulthood and can occur at any time of the day. The polysomnographic hallmark of narcolepsy is sleep-onset REM (SOREM). Whereas the normal REM latency is about 90 minutes, patients with narcolepsy often have a REM latency of less than 15 minutes. Narcolepsy occurs in about four of 10,000 people and has a definite familial basis. Studies have shown that 80–95% of patients with classic narcolepsy are positive for the HLA-DR2 antigen, depending on their ethnic background. The treatment of narcolepsy usually depends on which symptoms are bothering the patient. Treatment of sleep attacks usually includes the use of stimulants such as methylphenidate (Ritalin) or pemoline (Cylert). The attacks of cataplexy may be decreased by tricyclic antidepressants in doses below those used for depression.

Reference: page 255

Answer 11.4. **A,D**

The syndrome of periodic limb movements (PLMs) consists of stereotypic periodic leg movements during sleep that may or may not result in arousals. While 10–12% of patients seen in sleep centers for insomnia complaints have PLMs as the etiology, only 2–3% of the patients presenting with excessive daytime sleepiness are found to have PLMs as the major cause of their sleepiness. Patients with excessive somnolence due to PLMs may or may not remember the awakenings during the night but almost never remember the leg movements. The diagnosis of PLM syndrome requires monitoring of leg EMGs. Leg movements may occur in one or both legs, and therefore monitoring of both legs is suggested. Treatment of PLM syndrome is usually with benzodiazepines, which suppress awakenings but not the PLMs. The most commonly chosen agent is clonazepam 0.5 mg taken a half hour before bedtime.

Reference: pages 255–256

Answer 11.5. **B**

Conditions known to predispose patients to sleep apnea include the male sex, increasing age, alcohol use, obesity, hypothyroidism, acromegaly, and hypnotic use. While hypertension is common in patients with obstructive sleep apnea, its presence does not predispose a patient to develop clinical sleep apnea.

Reference: page 256

Answer 11.6. **A, C**

Polysomnography of patient with OSA syndrome reveals repetitive obstructive apneas and hypopneas. Apneas are followed by resumption of air flow, which usually coincides with evidence of arousal and often movement. During apnea the chest and abdomen move in a paradoxical manner. The heart rate usually slows during the apnea and then speeds up during the postapnea arousal. An increase in systolic blood pressure is associated with each obstructive apnea.

Reference: pages 257–258

Answer 11.7. **A, B, D**

The degree of arterial oxygen desaturation in patients with OSA is not necessarily correlated with the apnea index and must be considered in assessing the severity of the disease. A study of factors determining the severity of desaturation found that (a) a lower baseline PO_2, (b) a greater percentage of sleep time spent in apnea, and (c) a smaller expiratory reserve volume, all tended to produce more severe desaturation.

Reference: page 258

Answer 11.8. **B, C**

The upper airway of OSA patients is abnormal even during wakefulness. The supraglottic resistance is increased, and a higher than normal percentage of the maximal upper-airway muscle tone is required to preserve airway patency. Studies of the upper airway in awake patients with OSA by various imaging techniques have shown smaller than normal upper airways. In patients with OSA there is a periodic fluctuation in neural drive to both the upper airway and muscles of respiration. The amount of drive falls with the return to sleep and the onset of apnea, rises during the terminal phase of apnea, and is high at apnea termination and in the early post-apneic ventilatory period. The magnitude of the stimulus for arousal appears to depend on the level of inspiratory effort (ventilatory drive), rather than the individual levels of PO_2 and PCO_2.

Reference: pages 258–259

Answer 11.9. **C**

The exact causes of the excessive daytime somnolence in the obstructive sleep apnea syndrome are still under investigation. Sleep fragmentation is probably the most important factor, although hypoxemia may also play a role. Oximetry monitoring alone may not reflect the severity of a patient's sleep disorder, as some patients will have profound arterial oxygen desaturation with only mild to moderate symptoms of daytime sleepiness. Cognitive impairment does appear to be more severe in patients with sleep apnea who have hypoxemia. Treatment with tracheostomy or nasal CPAP frequently results in long periods of stages 3, 4, and REM on the first night when airway obstruction is prevented, and a rapid improvement in daytime alertness in many patients.

Reference: page 259

Answer 11.10. **A, D**

With nocturnal oxygen therapy, oxygenation usually improves, but the frequency of respiratory events usually decreases only slightly or remains unchanged; oxygen therapy does not improve the sleep latency on MSLT testing. No long-term studies have shown an improvement in morbidity or mortality with oxygen therapy. It may, however, improve cor pulmonale or arrhythmias associated with nocturnal desaturation in selected patients.

Reference: page 260

Answer 11.11.   **All are correct**

The main difficulty with nasal CPAP therapy is the problem with patient compliance; long-term compliance is at best around 60%. Nasal CPAP can dramatically reduce symptoms of daytime sleepiness and has also been shown to increase the sleep latency on MSLT testing. Studies have shown a decrease in mortality when patients with obstructive sleep apnea were treated with nasal CPAP. Treatment with nasal CPAP has also been shown to be effective in patients with obesity hypoventilation syndrome and may normalize the daytime PCO_2 in many patients.

Reference: pages 261–262

Answer 11.12.   **C, D**

In patients with CSA associated with periodic breathing, the normal fluctuations of breathing at sleep onset are exaggerated and persistent due to an instability in the ventilatory control and feedback systems. Factors predisposing to such instability include a high ventilatory response to hypoxia and hypercapnia, awake hypoxia and hypercapnia, a long circulation time (delayed feedback), and low oxygen stores.

Reference: page 263

Answer 11.13.   **A - True; B, C, D - False**

Patients with hypercapnic CSA usually have evidence of abnormalities in awake ventilatory control, neuromuscular weakness, or an abnormality in chest wall compliance. These patients usually present with episodes of hypercapnic respiratory failure and cor pulmonale. Morning headaches and daytime sleepiness are common. The degree of arterial oxygen desaturation tends to be severe, especially during REM sleep. The most effective therapy is nocturnal positive-pressure ventilation via a nasal mask or tracheostomy.

Reference: pages 263–264

Answer 11.14.   **A, C, D**

Studies in normal persons have shown that the best pulmonary function occurs at 4:00 PM and the worst at 4:00 AM. This fluctuation is even more pronounced in asthmatics. Nocturnal falls in circulating epinephrine and corticosteroids and increases in histamine and vagal tone may be important in the occurrence of nocturnal asthma. A recent study suggests that patients with significant worsening of lung function at night have a circadian influx of effector cells into the lung, with a significant increase in neutrophils and eosinophils in bronchoalveolar lavage done at 4:00 AM. Although theophylline could potentially disturb sleep quality, therapy with sustained-action theophylline was shown to be more effective than long-acting inhaled β-agonists in preventing nocturnal asthma.

Reference: page 265

Answer 11.15.   **A, B, D**

Patients with COPD may exhibit nocturnal desaturations with or without evidence of obstructive apnea. The episodes of profound desaturation seen during stage REM are usually associated with periods of hypopnea in which tidal volume is reduced but respiratory rate is essentially unchanged. Patients with CO_2 retention or resting hypoxia are more likely to exhibit severe desaturation. No study has documented that supplemental nocturnal oxygen will decrease mortality or morbidity in patients with desaturation confined to REM sleep. The group of patients with both COPD and OSA tend to have more severe cardiopulmonary sequelae than those with equivalent amounts of sleep apnea.

Reference: pages 266–267

chapter 12

Pulmonary Thromboembolism and Other Vascular Diseases

QUESTIONS

Question 12.1. **Which of the following are true or false regarding pulmonary thromboembolism and infarction of the lung?**

A. The frequency of thromboembolism associated with cardiac disease is higher than with urologic and obstetric patients combined.
B. Disorders associated with an increased frequency of pulmonary thromboembolism include antithrombin III deficiency, dysfibrinogenemia, antiphospholipid syndrome, and factor VII deficiency.
C. Autopsies reveal that about 30% of pulmonary emboli cause a pulmonary infarction.
D. Death from pulmonary thromboembolism still occurs in about 25% of patients after diagnosis despite adequate treatment.

Question 12.2. **Regarding the pathophysiologic mechanisms resulting from pulmonary artery obstruction from thromboembolism, which statements are true or false?**

A. A reduction in alveolar PCO_2 contributes to the development of local lung constriction.
B. Local surfactant activity begins to increase within 24 hours of the embolic event.
C. The mean pulmonary artery pressure systematically increases when 30% or more of the pulmonary vasculature is occluded by emboli.
D. Alveolar dead space increases as the result of local lung constriction.
E. Pulmonary artery pressures increase with pulmonary emboli while right ventricular work remains constant.

Question 12.3. **Regarding the clinical manifestations of pulmonary thromboembolism, which of the following are true or false?**

A. Perfusion defects by perfusion lung scans persist for 6 months in about one-fourth of patients with pulmonary emboli.
B. Leg swelling is the most common symptom associated with pulmonary emboli.
C. Large A waves in the jugular venous pulse and a loud P_2 component of the second heart sound are characteristic findings.
D. An $S_1Q_3T_3$ pattern on the electrocardiogram suggests pulmonary thromboembolism.
E. Fibrin degradation products in the serum are reduced in 90% of patients with angiographically proven pulmonary emboli.

Question 12.4. **Using the criteria of the PIOPED (prospective investigation of pulmonary embolism diagnosis) study, match the statements below with the probability based upon the ventilation/perfusion scan.**

1. One moderate segmental perfusion defect without corresponding ventilation defects or abnormalities on chest films.

2. One large segmental perfusion defect and two or more moderate defects without corresponding ventilation defects or abnormalities on chest films.

3. Four or more moderate segmental perfusion defects without corresponding ventilation defects or abnormalities on chest films.

4. Single or multiple small (<25% of a segment) segmental perfusion defects with a normal chest film.

5. Corresponding ventilation/perfusion defects and parenchymal opacities in lower lung zones on chest films.

6. Multiple matched ventilation/perfusion defects, regardless of size, with a normal chest film.

A. High probability
B. Intermediate probability
C. Low probability

Question 12.5. **Regarding ventilation/perfusion scans and pulmonary angiography, which statement is NOT true?**

A. Patients with pulmonary thromboembolism who are properly diagnosed and treated have a mortality of <10%.
B. A high clinical suspicion along with a low probability ventilation/perfusion scan still carries a 40% likelihood of a pulmonary embolus.
C. A reduction in perfusion as demonstrated by a Technetium-99 m lung scan is specific but not sensitive for diagnosing pulmonary thromboembolism.
D. With a low probability ventilation/perfusion scan and a high clinical suspicion of a pulmonary embolus, the physician should consider a pulmonary arteriogram despite negative impedance plethysmography (IPG) and Doppler ultrasound studies of the legs.

Question 12.6. **An 80-year-old woman sustains a hip fracture while falling at home. She is admitted to the hospital and is scheduled for a total hip replacement. Which of the following regimens is acceptable for prophylaxis of postoperative thromboembolism?**

A. Subcutaneous heparin every 12 hr starting 2 hours preoperatively.
B. Warfarin 1 mg per day beginning postoperatively until discharge.
C. Intermittent pneumatic compression devices with elastic stockings on the lower extremities.
D. Low dose warfarin at 2 mg per day.

Question 12.7. **Which statement below is correct regarding the treatment of deep venous thrombosis?**

A. Heparin is the drug of choice in acute thrombosis and works by inhibiting factors II, VII, IX, and X.
B. Thrombolytic therapy for deep venous thrombosis includes streptokinase, with effectiveness as high as 90% when used less than 10 days from presentation.

C. The incidence of major bleeding complications when using thrombolytic agents for deep venous thrombosis is over 10% higher than heparin alone.

D. Coumarin derivatives are typically initiated after 5–7 days of heparin when treating deep venous thrombosis with a target INR of 1 to 2.

Question 12.8. **A 75-year-old man with prostate cancer develops acute dyspnea. His heart rate is 115, respiratory rate 28, and blood pressure 100/50. His chest film shows mild hyperinflation with a prominent right pulmonary artery. His arterial pH is 7.45, $PaCO_2$ 30, and PaO_2 55, on room air. A ventilation/perfusion lung scan is reported as high probability. Following therapeutic heparinization, he develops worsening hypotension and respiratory arrest. Which statement below best describes this patient's clinical course?**

A. Emergency surgical embolectomy is indicated, with a success rate of 80%.

B. Thrombolytic therapy is routinely employed in patients with massive pulmonary emboli and has shown to decrease mortality by about 25%

C. Vena cava filter insertion is effective, with pulmonary emboli recurring in about 10% of patients following insertion.

D. The mortality rate for patients with the above clinical findings is about 20%.

Question 12.9. **Clinical findings in chronic thromboembolic pulmonary hypertension include all of the following EXCEPT:**

A. As many as 20% of patients will have deficiencies of antithrombin III or proteins C or S.

B. Unlike patients with chronic thromboembolism, patients with primary pulmonary hypertension will usually have a normal perfusion scan with only the pulmonary arteriogram confirming the diagnosis.

C. Late ECG findings of pulmonary hypertension due to recurrent emboli may include right axis deviation, right ventricular hypertrophy, and T-wave inversion.

D. On physical exam, there is usually jugular venous distention, hepatomegaly, leg edema, a loud P_2, and a murmur of tricuspid insufficiency late in the disease.

Question 12.10. **Which statement below is NOT true regarding embolism to the lungs by substances other than thromboemboli?**

A. Septic emboli should be treated with both antibiotics and anticoagulants.

B. Evidence that fat emboli may exist is found when fat stained by oil red O is present in about 60% of BAL specimens.

C. Amniotic fluid embolism is treated with corticosteroids and low dose heparin.

D. Air emboli may be suspected if angioedema of the face or neck and/or livedo reticularis is present; it is treated by positioning the patient in the left lateral decubitus position.

Question 12.11. **Regarding pulmonary hypertension (PH), which of the following statements is correct?**

A. Precapillary PH caused by increased flow conditions may be noted on chest films by decreased vascular markings in the peripheral 2 cm of the lungs.

B. Primary PH has mean pulmonary artery pressures greater than 30 mm Hg during exercise with elevated pulmonary artery wedge pressures.

C. Systemic lupus erythematosus is the most common connective tissue disease associated with PH.

D. In PH associated with living at high altitudes (Monge's disease), affected individuals will have a decreased sensitivity to carbon dioxide.

Question 12.12.   **Postcapillary pulmonary hypertension results largely from cardiac or pulmonary venous abnormalities. Which statement regarding this condition is NOT true?**

A.   Common causes of postcapillary pulmonary hypertension include left ventricular failure and mitral valve disease.

B.   Postcapillary pulmonary hypertension is manifest by orthopnea, dyspnea, and occasionally paroxysmal nocturnal dyspnea as a result of pulmonary edema.

C.   An anomalous pulmonary venous return results in precapillary pulmonary hypertension.

D.   Postcapillary pulmonary hypertension may result from an atrial myxoma with symptoms frequently relieved by changes in posture.

Question 12.13.   **The clinical manifestations of pulmonary hypertension vary depending on the disease process. Which statement below is NOT true?**

A.   Physical findings include Raynaud's phenomenon in 10%, however clubbing does not occur in primary pulmonary hypertension.

B.   Chest films often show a small aorta with large main and hilar pulmonary arteries and pruning of the peripheral vessels.

C.   In veno-occlusive disease there is evidence of increased bronchovascular markings and Kerley B lines while in classic pulmonary hypertension there is not.

D.   Pulmonary function test are not helpful in the evaluation of pulmonary hypertension.

Question 12.14.   **Which statements are True/False regarding the treatment and prognosis of pulmonary hypertension?**

A.   Chronic warfarin therapy has been shown to improve survival in patients with primary pulmonary hypertension.

B.   About 60% of patients respond to oral vasodilator therapy, but they still have a 5-year mortality of 50%.

C.   Continuous prostacyclin infusion is used in some patients with proven long-term benefit.

D.   Primary pulmonary hypertension patients may benefit from a double lung transplant, but not a single lung transplant.

E.   A reasonable goal with therapy is to reduce the pulmonary vascular resistance by 50%.

Question 12.15.   **A 60-year-old man with a 100 pack year smoking history is diagnosed with end stage emphysema. His physical exam demonstrates lower extremity edema and engorged jugular veins. He admits to increasing dyspnea over the last 3 months. An echocardiogram notes a left ventricular ejection fraction of 50% with an enlarged right ventricle and pulmonary arteries, and moderate tricuspid regurgitation. There is no evidence of myocardial ischemia. Which of the following statements is correct?**

A.   Of patients with COPD, approximately 50% of those older than 50 years develop pulmonary hypertension, with resistance measurements often greater than 550 dynes-second-cm^{-5}.

B.   This man's physical exam may also demonstrate a soft P_2 component of the second heart sound and an S_3 gallop.

C.   This patient's pulmonary artery trunks would measure about 10 to 12 mm on a standard posteroanterior chest film.

D. The treatment of choice is diuretics and digitalis for his apparent cardiac decompensation.

ANSWERS

Answer 12.1. **A, B - True; C, D - False**

Thrombus formation is related to blood stasis, hypercoagulable states, and vessel wall damage. Pulmonary emboli originate most often from veins of the deep femoral and pelvic systems, and from the right atrium. Risk factors are numerous (see Table 12.2, page 272, *Chest Medicine,* 3rd edition). Studies indicate that thromboembolism in cardiac patients may reach 40% in frequency while urologic (25% frequency) and obstetric (3% frequency) diseases combined are associated with fewer. Orthopedic procedures still account for the highest frequency, just under 70% in some series. Treatment of thrombus formation after diagnosis results in death in less than 10%, which makes a strong clinical suspicion paramount in decreasing morbidity and mortality. Less than 10% of pulmonary emboli cause a pulmonary infarction. Antithrombin III deficiency, dysfibrinogenemia, antiphospholipid (high anticardiolipin antibodies) syndrome, and factor VII deficiency are strongly associated with an increased frequency of thrombus formation.

Reference: pages 272, 273

Answer 12.2. **A, D - True; B, C, E - False**

Respiratory consequences of pulmonary artery obstruction from an embolus include an increase in alveolar dead space, pneumoconstriction, and loss of surfactant. There is a reduction in $PACO_2$ in the embolic segment leading to lung constriction and a subsequent increase in dead space. Within 24 hours of pulmonary artery occlusion, surfactant levels decrease, leading to alveolar collapse and associated atelectasis. More than 50% of the pulmonary vasculature must be occluded before increases in mean pulmonary artery pressure are significant. Large pulmonary artery emboli result in increases in pulmonary artery resistance and work of the right ventricle. The capacity for accommodation of the right ventricle to acute pressure loads is limited due to its thin muscle layer, which may lead to failure and cardiovascular collapse.

Reference: pages 273, 274

Answer 12.3. **C, D - True; A, B, E - False**

With pulmonary thromboemboli, dyspnea is the most common symptom and is found in about 75% of patients. Patients may have large A waves, an S_3 gallop, and a loud P_2 component of the second heart sound. An ECG may show an $S_1Q_3T_3$ pattern; however, the ECG is frequently normal except for tachycardia. Perfusion defects by perfusion lung scans remain in only 10% of patients after 6 weeks. The fibrinolytic system usually rapidly resolves the thrombi in survivors with more than 90% of patients demonstrating increased fibrin degradation products in the serum early in the disease course.

Reference: pages 275, 276

Answer 12.4. **1 - B, 2 - A, 3 - A, 4 - C, 5 - B, 6 - C**

The PIOPED study to categorized patients into groups of high, intermediate, and low probability based on ventilation/perfusion scan results and the associated clinical findings. One large segmental defect and two or more moderate defects, or four or more moderate segmental perfusion defects without corresponding ventilation defects or abnormalities on chest films, constitutes high probability for a pulmonary embolus. Intermediate probability includes up to two large segmental perfusion defects without corresponding ventilation defects or abnormal chest films, or corresponding ventilation/perfusion defects and parenchymal opacities in the lower lung zone on a chest film. A low probability scan includes single or multiple small segmental perfusion defects, or multiple matched ventilation/perfusion defects with a normal chest film. A complete listing of the PIOPED criteria is shown in Table 12.5.

Reference: page 278

Answer 12.5.   **C**

Perfusion scans of the lungs commonly involve technetium-99m-labeled albumin which is trapped in the pulmonary capillaries. The detection of the γ-emitting isotope is highly sensitive but lacks specificity as a result of the many possible causes of reduced regional pulmonary blood flow. Patients have a <10% mortality when properly treated. Pulmonary emboli occur in about 40% of patients with a low probability ventilation/perfusion scans when there is a strong clinical suspicion of thromboembolism. Therefore, physicians should consider an arteriogram in these patients even if an IPG or Doppler ultrasound is normal.

Reference: pages 277–279

Answer 12.6.   **D**

Orthopedic surgeries involving the hip are at the greatest risk for venous thromboembolism with up to an 80% incidence in some series. Current prophylaxis recommendations include low dose warfarin, 2 mg every day, or at a dose to keep the INR at 2–3. Low molecular weight heparin or adjusted dose heparin (aPTT 31–36) are increasingly recommended alternatives. General surgery patients less than 40 years old undergoing surgeries lasting less than 30 minutes typically can benefit from early ambulation alone. A more complete listing of prophylaxis indications is shown in Table 12.7.

Reference: page 281

Answer 12.7.   **B**

For acute deep venous thrombosis, heparin is the treatment of choice. Heparin inactivates thrombin, factors Xa and IXa by binding antithrombin III. Coumarin derivatives act by inhibiting coagulation factors II, VII, IX, and X as well as proteins C and S. Current recommendations are to initiate warfarin on day 1 or 2 to decrease the duration of heparin and hospital stay, with a target INR of 2–3. The incidence of major bleeding complications associated with the thrombolytic agents is no greater than heparin and warfarin alone. Streptokinase is best used if therapy is initiated before 5–10 days from presentation, with thrombolysis of existing clot in 90% of patients. The thrombin time is followed to measure the effectiveness of the thrombolytic infusion.

Reference: pages 281–283

Answer 12.8.   **D**

Massive pulmonary emboli typically result in hypoxia and hypotension and may occur as a result of a hypercoagulable state such as that associated with prostate cancer. Surgical embolectomy is used only for extreme cases and carries a mortality rate from 50% to more than 90%. Thrombolytic agents have been shown to reduce clot size but have not been shown to increase survival. Vena cava filters are indicated when massive pulmonary emboli have occurred and clots remain in the proximal deep venous system. Filters are also used in patients who have contraindications to anticoagulants or thrombolytics. Emboli recur in <2% of patients with filters in place. The mortality from pulmonary emboli when shock is evident is about 20%.

Reference: pages 283, 284

Answer 12.9.   **A**

Classical late findings of elevated pulmonary artery pressure from chronic thromboembolism include elevated right heart pressures manifest on physical exam by hepatomegaly, lower extremity edema, a loud P_2, and a systolic murmur of tricuspid insufficiency. Electrocardiograms may demonstrate right axis deviation, right ventricular hypertrophy and T-wave inversion. With thromboembolism, the perfusion scan is abnormal while in primary pulmonary hypertension, the scan is normal or shows only patchy subsegmental defects. A pulmonary arterial angiogram may confirm the diagnosis by showing intraluminal bands, webs, intimal irregularities, or vascular narrowing and obstruction. Less than 1% of affected patients will demonstrate a hypercoagulable state with antithrombin III or proteins C and S deficiencies.

Reference: page 284

Answer 12.10.   **C**

Septic emboli may occur in intravenous drug users, following gynecologic-obstetric procedures, and after any arterial/venous cannulation. Evidence supports the use of both antibiotics and anticoagulants for optimal treatment. Fat emboli, usually associated with long bone fractures, may be suspected if patients develop a petechial rash on the chest and arms. BAL specimens demonstrate fat by oil red O stain. Embolism of amniotic fluid carries a mortality of 80–90%, with treatment only being supportive. Corticosteroids and heparin are of no proven benefit. Air emboli can be fatal in large boluses because of obstruction to the pulmonary blood flow. Patients should be moved to the left lateral decubitus position immediately to avoid as much air entering the right ventricle as possible. Patients may develop angioedema of the face and neck with livedo reticularis. Seizures, strokes, or cardiovascular collapse may occur suddenly.

Reference: pages 284–287

Answer 12.11.   **D**

High flow states leading to pulmonary hypertension (PH), such as congenital left to right shunts, will cause an enlargement of all of the precapillary pulmonary vessels, causing vessels in the peripheral lung to become visible. In primary PH, mean pulmonary pressures are greater than 30 mm Hg with exercise; patients have normal pulmonary artery wedge pressures. Scleroderma is the connective tissue disease most often associated with PH, which occurs in up to 60% of patients. Chronic mountain sickness is the result of prolonged living at high altitude, with resulting PH. Affected individuals have a decreased sensitivity to carbon dioxide, and their alveolar carbon dioxide tensions are higher, resulting in pulmonary artery vasoconstriction.

Reference: pages 288, 289

Answer 12.12.   **C**

Postcapillary pulmonary hypertension most commonly results from failure of the left ventricle along with mitral valve disease, myxoma or thrombus of the left atrium, congenital stenosis at the origin of the pulmonary veins, mediastinal granulomas and neo-plasms, idiopathic veno-occlusive disease, and anomalous pulmonary venous return. Patients will have symptoms of pulmonary edema including orthopnea, dyspnea, and occasionally paroxysmal nocturnal dyspnea and frothy sputum. Improvement in symptoms often follows treatment of the inducing cause.

References: pages 289, 290

Answer 12.13.   **D**

The clinical findings of pulmonary hypertension vary, with evidence of pulmonary edema (increased bronchovascular markings, Kerley B lines) occurring only with post-capillary disorders. Raynaud's phenomenon may occur in 10% of patients, and clubbing does not occur in primary pulmonary hypertension (but may in some congenital cardiac shunts and pulmonary hypertension associated with the collagen vascular diseases). Chest films often show large pulmonary arteries with an abrupt cutoff of peripheral vessels (pruning). Pulmonary function tests are useful to determine the amount of obstruction a patient may have, as many chronic COPD patients develop pulmonary hypertension in the late stages of their disease.

References: pages 290, 291

Answer 12.14.   **A - True; B, C, D, E - False**

Most patients with primary pulmonary hypertension follow a progressive and fatal course. Treatment consists of oxygen, vasodilators, and anticoagulation, with chronic use of warfarin showing increases in survival. Only about one-fourth of patients respond to therapy, however responders have a 5-year survival of 94%. Chronic use of continuous prostacyclin may result in tachyphylaxis. Reductions in the pulmonary vascular resistance of at least 20% will help off-load the right ventricle and avoid further heart failure. Single and double lung transplants as well as heart/lung transplants have been used for primary pulmonary hypertension.

References: pages 292, 293

Answer 12.15.   **A**

Cor pulmonale refers to the enlargement of the right ventricle secondary to disorders affecting lung structure or function. This man's end-stage emphysema has led to a reduction in the cross-sectional pulmonary vascular bed and secondary right heart decompensation. About 50% of patients with COPD over 50 years of age will develop pulmonary hypertension. On chest films, the pulmonary arteries may measure >16 mm on the right and >19 mm on the left, suggesting high vascular pressures. A P_2 may be palpable, and an S_4 is often apparent. Oxygen is the initial choice of therapy, often followed by diuresis occurring after increases in cardiac output by lowering the pulmonary vascular resistance. Digitalis has little role in the treatment of cor pulmonale.

References: pages 293–295

chapter 13

Diffuse Interstitial and Alveolar Inflammatory Diseases

QUESTIONS

Question 13.1. **A 60-year-old man, without a significant past medical history, complains of gradually increasing shortness of breath. He admits to an occasional dry cough, fatigue, and a 10 lb weight loss. He has dry (Velcro-type) crackles in both bases without jugular venous distention or peripheral edema. There is mild clubbing of his fingers. A chest radiograph shows a diffuse reticular pattern prominent in the lower lung fields. His arterial pH 7.40, PaCo$_2$ 38 mm Hg, and PaO$_2$ 58 mm Hg breathing room air. There is no history of occupational or infectious disease exposure. Which statement below would be most consistent with this patient's diagnosis?**

A. With advanced disease, pulmonary function tests demonstrate a reduction in total lung capacity and residual volume without significant changes in diffusing capacity.
B. Transbronchial biopsies with a simultaneous bronchoalveolar lavage will yield the diagnosis in the majority of patients with this disease.
C. The use of ^{67}Ga gallium citrate isotope is helpful in correlating disease activity and is used routinely to follow the disease.
D. The erythrocyte sedimentation rate (ESR) is elevated in most cases, with associated elevations of circulating immunoglobulin levels in 30% and cryoimmunoglobulins in as many as 40% of cases.

Question 13.2. **Regarding idiopathic pulmonary fibrosis (IPF), which statement below best describes the associated histology and staging of disease activity?**

A. Factors which give the patient a more favorable prognosis include male sex, a gradual onset, and increases in inflammatory cells, especially polymorphonuclear granulocytes (PMNs).
B. Alveolitis, thus desquamative interstitial pneumonitis (DIP), is diagnosed when macrophages, type II pneumocytes, PMNs and eosinophils are found in the alveolar spaces.
C. Biopsies, transbronchial or open lung, demonstrate the cellular pathology used in staging, while bronchoalveolar lavage (BAL) material does not correlate with the ongoing interstitial process.
D. Biopsies that contain PMNs, eosinophils, and especially lymphocytes, correlate with a poor response to corticosteroid therapy.
E. The neutrophil is thought to be responsible for the acute injury that is perpetuated into a chronic phase due to continued activation or poor regulation.

Question 13.3. **The treatment of idiopathic pulmonary fibrosis (IPF) may include the use of immunosuppressive drugs. Which statement below best describes prognosis and response to therapy?**

A. Desquamative alveolar stages of IPF have about a 20% rate of spontaneous remission without the use of an immunosuppressive agent.

B. Prednisone is a mainstay of therapy and is usually given at doses of 1.0 mg/kg/day for 1 year before reassessing its efficacy.

C. The risk of developing lung cancer is no greater in patients with IPF than in the general population.

D. Recently, the use of colchicine had been shown to worsen the fibrosis seen in IPF.

Question 13.4. **Regarding the diagnosis of bronchiolitis obliterans organizing pneumonia (BOOP), which statement is *not* true?**

A. Histologic characteristics of BOOP include polyploid masses of granulation tissue in the lumens of small airways, alveolar ducts, and some alveoli.

B. Patients present with a cough or flu-like illness for several weeks, with crackles on physical examination; chest radiographs show a "ground-glass" appearance with localized air space densities in the majority of patients.

C. Pulmonary function tests reveal an obstructive ventilatory impairment in the majority patients.

D. Corticosteroid treatment is efficacious, with complete clinical and physiologic recovery in as many as 65% of patients.

Question 13.5. **A 25-year-old woman comes to your office with complaints of increasing dyspnea, mild joint aches, a dry cough with pleuritic chest pain, and a new rash on her face. She describes a fullness in her right chest with the inability to take a deep breath. She has no infectious or occupational exposures. On physical examination, she has decreased breath sounds in her right base with basilar crackles bilaterally. A chest radiograph reveals a small right pleural effusion with some basilar atelectasis. Her oxygen saturation is 90%, hemoglobin 10 g/dL, and ANA titer 1:1024. Her HIV test is negative. Which statement below concerning the diagnosis and treatment is true?**

A. Interstitial lung disease with patchy fibrosis is the most common intrathoracic manifestation of this disease.

B. The finding of LE cells in her pleural fluid is diagnostic of her disease.

C. Microthrombi appear to be the most likely cause when infiltrates are found on a chest radiograph.

D. Patients demonstrate digital clubbing on physical examination and an obstructive ventilatory impairment on spirometry.

E. Patients with this disease have not demonstrated an increase in pulmonary emboli when the antiphospholipid antibody syndrome is present.

Question 13.6. **Which of the following is not a pleuropulmonary manifestation of systemic lupus erythematosus (SLE)?**

A. Pulmonary vasculitis
B. Acute lupus pneumonitis
C. Diffuse alveolar hemorrhage
D. Diffuse interstitial lung disease
E. Pleural effusion

Question 13.7.   **Which one of the following statements regarding pleural disease in rheumatoid arthritis (RA) is correct?**

A. The pleural fluid glucose is normal.
B. Empyema is the most common cause of a pleural effusion in RA.
C. Pleurisy has a predilection for females with RA.
D. Pleural disease is the most common thoracic complication of RA.

Question 13.8.   **Which statements concerning interstitial lung disease (ILD) in patients with rheumatoid arthritis (RA) are TRUE or FALSE?**

A. This complication of RA has a predilection for men.
B. Pulmonary function tests are more sensitive than the chest radiograph for detecting ILD in rheumatoid arthritis.
C. Of patients with RA and ILD, 50% have subcutaneous nodules.
D. The lung infiltrates are most marked in the apices of the lungs.

Question 13.9.   **Which of the following statements are TRUE or FALSE regarding intrapulmonary (necrobiotic) nodules in patients with rheumatoid arthritis?**

A. These nodules have a predilection for the lower lung zones.
B. Their identification in the lungs may precede joint manifestations of RA.
C. Spontaneous pneumothorax may occur in such patients.
D. Their occurrence is more common in men with RA.
E. Pathologically, these nodules are identical to the subcutaneous nodules in RA.

Question 13.10.   **A 53-year-old woman has complaints of numbness, tightness, and redness of her hands on exposure to cold. Further history reveals recurrent "chest colds" and evidence of gastroesophageal reflux disease. She is on no medications, does not smoke, and has no contributory past medical history. Her chest film shows an interstitial reticular pattern in both bases with mild pleural thickening. Which one of the following statements is correct?**

A. Penicillamine therapy has resulted in improvement in DLCO in this disease.
B. The patient will demonstrate a reduction in lung volumes as the most common early manifestation of lung involvement.
C. A trial of prednisone 0.5–1 mg/kg/day is indicated.
D. With γ-interferon therapy the 5-year survival after the detection of lung disease is greater than 50%.
E. Pleural disease is more common in this disease than interstitial lung disease.

Question 13.11.   **Which of the following statements are TRUE or FALSE regarding patients with scleroderma (progressive systemic sclerosis)?**

A. The lung is the most common visceral organ involved with this disease.
B. The most common chest radiograph abnormality is an interstitial reticular pattern, particularly affecting the lung apices.
C. Pulmonary vascular disease develops as an extension of the interstitial lung disease in this disorder.
D. The 5-year survival rate following detection of lung disease in patients with scleroderma is 70%.

Question 13.12.   **A 60-year-old woman presents with gradual onset of dyspnea and cough; her chest radiograph shows diffuse pulmonary infiltrates, most prominent in the lung bases. The patient also complains of increased weakness and pain in her** proximal muscle groups. On physical examination, she has basilar crackles and ery-thematous skin lesions on her abdomen and lower extremities. Which statement below best describes this patient's disease process?

A. Pleural disease is a prominent feature of this disease.
B. The histopathology of this disease process includes bronchiolitis obliterans orga-nizing pneumonia and usual interstitial pneumonia.
C. The pulmonary disease only rarely precedes the skin and muscle manifestations of this disease.
D. Corticosteroids do not cause significant disease remission.

Question 13.13. **Which of the following statements are TRUE or FALSE regarding polymyositis/dermatomyositis (PM-DM)?**

A. PM-DM includes a group of diffuse inflammatory and degenerating disorders of striated muscle that cause symmetrical weakness and atrophy of distal muscle groups.
B. The disease is twice as common in females as in males.
C. It shows one peak age incidence in the fifth and sixth decades.
D. Pleural disease is common in PM-DM.
E. In contrast to rheumatoid arthritis and systemic lupus erythematosus, primary in-terstitial lung disease does not complicate PM-DM.

Question 13.14. **Which of the following statements are TRUE or FALSE regarding Wegener's granulomatosis (WG)?**

A. WG is twice as common in females as males.
B. Sinusitis is a common paranasal manifestation of WG.
C. Over 60% of patients with pulmonary involvement in WG present with hemopty-sis.
D. Although classically patients with pulmonary involvement in WG have a restrictive ventilatory defect, more than 50% of these patients also have an obstructive defect.
E. A positive p-ANCA titer is diagnostic of WG.

Question 13.15. **Which statements are TRUE/FALSE regarding the clinical features of Wegener's granulomatosis (WG)?**

A. Total complement levels are decreased in most patients with WG.
B. The perinuclear form of antineutrophil cytoplasm antibody (p-ANCA) is more spe-cific for WG than the c-ANCA pattern.
C. Patients typically exhibit mild hyperglobulinemia, particularly of the IgA fraction.
D. There is a good correlation between disease activity and ANCA titers.
E. Chest radiographic abnormalities are present in all patients with WG.

Question 13.16. **Which of the following statements regarding the treatment and prognosis of Wegener's granulomatosis (WG) is/are correct?**

A. Untreated, WG pursues a rapidly fatal course with a mean survival time of ap-proximately 5 months.
B. Corticosteroids do not significantly alter the long-term prognosis, although this therapy increases mean survival by 12 months.
C. Cytoxan (cyclophosphamide) therapy is associated with an approximately 50% re-lapse rate in WG.
D. Due to its low propensity to cause irreversible ovarian damage, methotrexate is con-traindicated in young women with WG.

Question 13.17.   **Which one of the following statements is correct regarding lymphomatoid granulomatosis (LYG)?**

A.   The female to male ratio is about 2:1 and most patients are in early middle age.
B.   Sinus and upper airway are the two most common extrathoracic sites of involvement in LYG.
C.   On the chest radiograph, the pulmonary lesions predominate in the upper lung fields peripherally, and they are usually bilateral.
D.   LYG resembles an indolent lymphoma and in many instances it progresses to an atypical disseminated lymphoproliferative disease.

Question 13.18.   **Which of the following statements are TRUE/FALSE regarding allergic angiitis (Churg-Strauss syndrome)?**

A.   Most patients with the Churg-Strauss syndrome will have an allergic background, often with asthma.
B.   The erythrocyte sedimentation rate and the degree of peripheral blood eosinophilia are good indicators of disease activity.
C.   Acutely, exudates from the lungs contain a predominance of eosinophilic leukocytes mixed with giant cells.
D.   Prednisone 1 mg/kg/day provides long-term remissions in most patients.
E.   Allergic angiitis and polyarteritis nodosa affect the pulmonary circulation in a similar manner.

Question 13.19.   **A 30-year-old man presents with massive hemoptysis resulting in respiratory failure and requiring mechanical ventilation. His chest radiograph reveals bilateral patchy alveolar filling infiltrates. His complete blood count shows a hemoglobin of 9 mg/dl and a white blood cell count of 10,000 cells/mm^3. Serum creatinine is 3.6 mg/dl and his urinalysis reveals 4+ red blood cells and proteinuria. His serum contains an elevated antiglomerular basement membrane (anti-GBM) antibody. There is no significant past medical history and he denies HIV risk factors. Which statement below is true regarding this patient?**

A.   The anemia associated with his disease is hemolytic in origin.
B.   The removal of the anti-GBM antibodies by plasmapheresis will lead to recovery of renal function.
C.   Long-term remissions are common with corticosteroid treatment alone.
D.   The disease is inactive when the antibody is not detected.

Question 13.20.   **Which of the following statements regarding Goodpasture's syndrome is/are correct?**

A.   There is a female predominance in the occurrence of this disease.
B.   Of all patients, 75% are between the ages of 17 and 27 years at the onset of the illness.
C.   Urinary findings are present on admission in 50% of patients, and these include proteinuria, microscopic hematuria, and less commonly, pyuria.
D.   Goodpasture's syndrome demonstrates a predilection for perihilar involvement; in contrast to the pulmonary congestion and edema of left ventricular failure, Kerley B lines and pleural effusions are not characteristic.

Question 13.21.   **Many similarities exist between Goodpasture's syndrome and idiopathic pulmonary hemosiderosis (IPH). Which of the following statement(s) are TRUE/FALSE concerning IPH and Goodpasture's?**

A. Goodpasture's syndrome is more likely than IPH to present clinically with hemoptysis.
B. Goodpasture's syndrome is characterized by circulating antiglomerular basement membrane antibodies while IPH has no identifiable abnormal antibodies.
C. IPH is not associated with coexisting renal disease while Goodpasture's syndrome always involves the kidneys.
D. Patients with Goodpasture's syndrome may have an elevated diffusion capacity by pulmonary function tests while in IPH the diffusion capacity is typically normal or low.
E. Prognostically, the disease remission rate is similar in IPH and Goodpasture's syndrome with or without the use of immunosuppressive therapy.

Question 13.22. **A 30-year-old man presents to the emergency room with respiratory distress. His arterial pH is 7.45, $PaCO_2$ 26 mm Hg, and PaO_2 50 mm Hg breathing room air. On physical examination he has scattered course crackles. A chest radiograph shows bilateral diffuse patchy and nodular infiltrates without pleural effusions. The patient is treated for pneumonia but fails to respond to antibiotics and is referred to you for bronchoscopy. Bronchial samples reveal a PAS-positive staining material noted to be proteinaceous and lipid rich. Methenamine-silver stains are negative. The physician should:**

A. Begin corticosteroids as it has been shown to be effective in this syndrome.
B. Expect an obstructive component on spirometry as a result of the proteinaceous material in peripheral airways.
C. Consider total lung lavage in the operating room.
D. Look for atypical mycobacteria as they are a common cause of infection in this syndrome.

Question 13.23. **Which of the following statements are TRUE or FALSE regarding bleomycin-induced lung disease?**

A. Occurrence of lung disease has not been shown to correlate with the dose of bleomycin administered.
B. Younger people are more subject to bleomycin pulmonary toxicity.
C. Simultaneous administration of thoracic radiation and bleomycin increases the likelihood of pulmonary toxicity.
D. Administration of high oxygen concentrations produces synergistic pulmonary toxicity with bleomycin.
E. In patients receiving bleomycin, hypersensitivity pulmonary toxicity can develop, and this entity is more amenable to improvement with corticosteroid therapy than other forms of bleomycin lung toxicity.

Question 13.24. **The therapeutic agents listed below may produce drug-induced pulmonary disease. MATCH the agent with the common associated pulmonary toxic reaction or clinical finding.**

1. Penicillamine
2. Gold salts, penicillamine, and sulfasalazine
3. Nitrofurantoin
4. Procainamide and hydralazine
5. Methotrexate

A. Associated with bronchiolitis obliterans
B. Associated with pulmonary-renal syndromes
C. Associated with pleuropulmonary lupus reactions

D. Increased incidence of hypersensitivity pneumonitis
E. Chronic toxicity associated with blood eosinophilia

Question 13.25.   **Which of the following drugs is not known to induce systemic lupus erythematosus (SLE)?**

A. Procainamide
B. Lidocaine
C. Hydralazine
D. Diphenylhydantoin
E. Sulfonamides

Question 13.26.   **Which of the following statements are TRUE/FALSE regarding amiodarone-induced pulmonary disease?**

A. Approximately 50% of patients receiving this antiarrhythmic agent develop lung disease.
B. Hypersensitivity pneumonitis can be induced by this drug.
C. Toxicity does not correlate with dose.
D. A diffusion capacity for carbon monoxide (DLCO) greater than 80% of pretreatment level virtually excludes amiodarone toxicity.

Question 13.27.   **A 26-year-old woman presents with a persistent cough and a 20 pound weight loss. Her chest radiograph reveals bilateral tracheal and hilar adenopathy with basilar interstitial markings. The angiotensin converting enzyme (ACE) level is elevated. Her other laboratory results are normal, and her PPD is nonreactive. She has no infectious or occupational exposures. Which statement below best applies to this patient?**

A. The hallmark of the immune response to this disease is a delayed type of hypersensitivity.
B. As many as 50% of patients with this disease will present with unilateral adenopathy.
C. Most patients will demonstrate an obstructive ventilatory impairment with normal diffusing capacity for carbon monoxide (DLCO).
D. The recovery of large numbers of neutrophils in the BAL fluid is a significant finding in many patients with this disease.
E. The majority of lymphocytes in BAL fluid can be identified as B cells.

Question 13.28.   **Which one of the following is not a complication of sarcoidosis?**

A. Uveitis
B. Neurologic signs
C. Cardiac arrhythmias
D. Hypocalcemia
E. Liver dysfunction

Question 13.29.   **Which of the following statements are TRUE/FALSE correct regarding sarcoidosis?**

A. Skin test anergy to common fungi and tuberculin antigens is a usual feature of active sarcoidosis.
B. Patients with both active and chronic forms of the disease can have fewer blood lymphocytes than normal.
C. Leukopenia appears in about 30% of patients.
D. Serum globulin levels are increased in about half of patients with active disease.

Question 13.30.   **Serum angiotensin converting enzyme (ACE) levels are increased in about half of patients with active sarcoidosis. In which of the following diseases is the serum ACE level not described to be elevated?**

A. Asbestosis
B. Systemic lupus erythematosus
C. Silicosis
D. Berylliosis
E. *Mycobacterium intracellulare* infection

Question 13.31.   **Match the lettered source of exposure to the numbered disease:**

1. Sequoiosis
2. Summer-type hypersensitivity
3. Suberosis
4. Farmer's lung
5. Bagassosis

A. Moldy cork dust
B. Moldy sugar cane fiber
C. Moldy hay
D. Moldy redwood dust
E. House dust or bird droppings

Question 13.32.   **Inhalation of a variety of organic dusts can cause hypersensitivity pneumonitis (or allergic alveolitis). Which statement below is true regarding this disease?**

A. Sensitization to an organic dust in the lungs is usually abrupt.
B. An immediate asthmatic-type reaction develops just after aerosol exposure to an antigen, and is characterized by air trapping and obstruction.
C. Digital clubbing is not associated with hypersensitivity pneumonitis.
D. Despite chronic aerosol exposures with subsequent restrictive ventilatory impairment, chest films remain normal in appearance.

Question 13.33.   **Which of the following is/are TRUE/FALSE regarding the findings in bronchoalveolar lavage (BAL) fluid in patients with chronic stages of hypersensitivity pneumonitis?**

A. Total protein is increased.
B. There is abnormal surfactant composition.
C. Large and foamy macrophages are recovered.
D. High polymorphonuclear leukocyte (PMN) counts are noted with low lymphocyte percentages.

Question 13.34.   **Which statements are TRUE/FALSE regarding the pathogenesis and treatment of hypersensitivity pneumonitis?**

A. The initial approach to treatment of hypersensitivity pneumonitis is administration of corticosteroids.
B. Bronchoalveolar fluid from these patients contains high numbers of lymphocytes and elevations in IgG and IgM.
C. In the acute stages of disease, there appears to be no increase in the number of eosinophils.
D. Skin testing with fungal hypersensitivity antigens is generally unreliable except for aspergillosis.

Question 13.35. **Which statements are TRUE/FALSE regarding the pulmonary eosinophilic syndrome?**

A. Simple pulmonary eosinophilia (Loeffler's pneumonia or PIE syndrome) is associated with parasitic infections and sulfonamide antibiotics.

B. Prolonged pulmonary eosinophilia commonly affects women, may not demonstrate blood eosinophilia, and has migrating infiltrates on chest films.

C. In tropical pulmonary eosinophilia, BAL fluid may contain antibodies to *Brugia malayi* with microfilaria identified in tissue nodules.

D. Two diseases associated with pulmonary eosinophilia and asthma are allergic bronchopulmonary aspergillosis and allergic angiitis with granulomatosis.

Question 13.36. **Regarding the eosinophilic granuloma syndrome [Histiocytosis X or Langerhans's cell granulomatosis (LCG)], which statements are TRUE/FALSE?**

A. LCG is called Hand-Schuller-Christian disease when lytic skull lesions, exophthalmos, and the pituitary are involved.

B. LCG typically affects young females who smoke.

C. A patient with LCG may classically present with a pneumothorax and diffuse micronodular densities and interstitial-appearing infiltrates on chest films.

D. Of patients with LCG, 20% will develop lytic bone lesions.

E. Corticosteroids are indicated in the initial treatment, and are effective in about 60% of patients.

ANSWERS

Answer 13.1.   **D**

Idiopathic pulmonary fibrosis, or cryptogenic fibrosing alveolitis, is manifested clinically by a nonproductive cough, a sensation of breathlessness, crackles on physical examination, and arterial hypoxemia. The average age at diagnosis is about 50 years. Almost all patients have a restrictive ventilatory impairment with a greater than 50% reduction in diffusing capacity. Chest radiographs reveal a diffuse bibasilar reticular pattern while high resolution CT scanning often demonstrates a "ground glass" appearance (see Fig. 13.2, page 307 in text). Transbronchial biopsies are usually performed first; however, they are inconclusive in the majority of IPF patients, necessitating the consideration of an open lung biopsy. Gallium scanning is inconsistent, and therefore not reliable for determining disease activity and response to therapy. The ESR is elevated in 90% of patients while studies have shown elevations in serum immunoglobulin levels in 30% and cryoimmunoglobulins in as many as 40% of cases.

Reference: pages 305–308

Answer 13.2.   **B**

Idiopathic pulmonary fibrosis is classified into various stages based upon histologic appearance. The acute alveolitis phase, or desquamative interstitial pneumonitis, is manifest by macrophages, type II pneumocytes, PMN's, and eosinophils in the alveolar spaces. The cellular material obtained by bronchoalveolar lavage (BAL) has been shown to correlate with the activity occurring in the interstitial spaces. Females, patients with an acute onset, and those whose BAL contains PMNs, eosinophils, and especially lymphocytes, tend to have a more favorable prognosis and response to corticosteroid therapy. The macrophage plays an important role in this immunologically mediated disease in the acute as well as the chronic phases due to continued activation or poor regulation. The inciting antigen in IPF is still unknown but is thought to possibly be a viral protein.

Reference: pages 309–310

Answer 13.3. **A**

Corticosteroids are the mainstay of treatment in idiopathic pulmonary fibrosis (IPF) and are initiated at doses of 1 mg/kg/day for 6–8 weeks, then tapered to 0.25 mg/kg/day for up to a year with periodic monitoring of pulmonary function tests and arterial blood gases. Other immunosuppressives used include cyclophosphamide, azathioprine, and penicillamine. Recently colchicine has been effective in some IPF patients; however, larger prospective trials are anticipated. Alveolitis, or the desquamative alveolar stages, have about a 20% rate of spontaneous remission whether immunosuppressives are used or not. Lung carcinoma has a 14-fold increased incidence in men and a 6-fold increased incidence in women with IPF.

Reference: pages 311–312

Answer 13.4. **C**

Bronchiolitis obliterans organizing pneumonia (BOOP), as opposed to bronchiolitis obliterans, demonstrates a restrictive ventilatory impairment with a decrease in diffusion capacity. Histologic specimens reveal granulation tissue in the alveolar ducts, lumens of small airways, and some alveoli. The presentation is usually with a nonproductive cough, malaise, and fatigue for several weeks. Chest radiographs will show a "ground-glass" appearance in most patients, with localized air space densities. Patients usually respond to corticosteroids, and will recover in a few months to years.

Reference: pages 312–313

Answer 13.5. **B**

Pleural disease is the most common intrathoracic manifestation of systemic lupus erythematosus. Effusions are usually bilateral and often are painful. The finding of LE cells in the pleural fluid is considered diagnostic; however, the finding of an elevated ANA titer in the pleural fluid and serum is helpful. The pleural fluid usually has a normal pH and glucose concentration (contrasted to rheumatoid pleural effusions). Infections, and not lupus pneumonitis, are the most common etiology associated with infiltrates in lupus patients. Digital clubbing is not a common physical finding, and patients demonstrate a restrictive ventilatory impairment. Often basilar atelectasis occurs due to diaphragmatic dysfunction. Patients with lupus have an increased risk of pulmonary emboli when circulating anticoagulant is present.

Reference: pages 313–315

Answer 13.6: **A**

Acute lupus pneumonitis, diffuse alveolar hemorrhage, diffuse interstitial lung disease, and pleural effusion are all well-recognized complications of SLE. However, pulmonary vasculitis is not a feature of SLE.

Reference: page 313

Answer 13.7. **D**

The pleural fluid glucose is characteristically low in RA, often markedly depressed. Empyema occurs rarely in patients with RA. Pleurisy has a predilection for males with

RA even though RA is more common in females. Pleural disease is the most common thoracic complication of RA.

Reference: page 315

Answer 13.8. **A, B, C-True; D-False**

Similar to pleural disease in patients with rheumatoid arthritis, ILD has a predilection for males. Only 2% of patients with RA have ILD on chest radiograph in large series, whereas 40% or more have some pulmonary function testing abnormalities. There is an association between subcutaneous nodules and ILD in patients with RA. The lung infiltrates are most marked in the bases of patients with ILD due to rheumatoid arthritis.

Reference: page 315

Answer 13.9. **B, C, D, E-True; A-False**

Intrapulmonary nodules in RA have predilection for the upper lung zones and male sex. Their identification may precede the joint manifestations of the disease. Usually peripheral in location, these lesions may induce a pneumothorax. They are pathologically identical to subcutaneous nodules in rheumatoid arthritis.

Reference: pages 315–316

Answer 13.10. **A**

Progressive systemic sclerosis (scleroderma) is a disorder of connective tissue resulting in fibrosis and vascular abnormalities. The lungs are second only to the esophagus in incidence of involvement. When lung disease is present, the 5-year survival is less than 50% despite treatment. Interstitial disease with subsequent honeycombing and cyst formation is the most common abnormality on chest films. A decrease in DLCO is the earliest pulmonary function abnormality, and usually precedes a reduction in lung volumes. Penicillamine has been shown to increase the DLCO in some cases while γ-interferon may improve the skin involvement and arterial oxygen tension. Corticosteroids are not helpful in the treatment of scleroderma lung disease.

Reference: pages 316–317

Answer 13.11. **A, B, C, D-False**

The esophagus is the most common visceral organ involved with scleroderma, followed by the lungs. The interstitial lung disease has a predilection for the bases. The pulmonary vascular disease in scleroderma is separate and distinct from interstitial lung manifestations. The 5-year survival rate is less than 50% following detection of lung disease.

Reference: pages 316–317

Answer 13.12. **B**

Polymyositis-dermatomyositis is an inflammatory and degenerative disorder of striated muscle with associated erythematous skin lesions. Pulmonary complications may precede, follow, or occur simultaneously with the other systemic signs and symptoms. Pleural disease is rare. Pathology includes bronchiolitis obliterans organizing pneumonia, usual interstitial pneumonia, diffuse alveolar damage, and pulmonary arteriolitis. Corticosteroids have caused remission in about 50% of patients. Significant problems include chronic aspiration due to a hypotonic esophagus and hypostatic pneumonia secondary to chest wall involvement.

Reference: pages 317–318

Answer 13.13.   **B-True; A, C, D, E-False**

Polymyositis-dermatomyositis (PM-DM) causes symmetrical weakness and atrophy of proximal muscle groups. The disease is twice as common in females as in males. There are two peak age incidences for PM-DM: the first decade and the fifth and sixth decades. In contrast to RA and SLE, pleural disease is uncommon in PM-DM; however, primary interstitial lung disease does complicate PM-DM in approximately 5% of patients.

Reference: page 317

Answer 13.14.   **B, D-True; A, C, E-False**

Wegener's granulomatosis (WG) is almost twice as frequent in males as in females. Sinusitis (67%) is the most common head and neck finding in WG, followed by otitis media (29%), rhinitis or nasal symptoms (22%), epistaxis (11%), ulcers (6%), and hearing impairment (6%). Only 18% of patients with WG noticed hemoptysis in Fauci's series. An obstructive defect as well as a restrictive defect is common in WG. c-ANCA, not p-ANCA, is considered specific for WG.

Reference: pages 318–320

Answer 13.15.   **C, D-True; A, B, E-False**

Wegener's granulomatosis (WG) features include necrotizing granulomatous vasculitis of the upper and lower respiratory tracts, glomerulonephritis, and variable degrees of small vessel vasculitis. The diffuse granular pattern of antineutrophil cytoplasm antibody (c-ANCA) is more specific for WG than the perinuclear pattern (p-ANCA), and titers closely correlate with disease activity. Normal or elevated complement levels with hyperglobulinemia of the IgA subtype are frequent. Chest radiograph abnormalities are present in three-fourths of affected patients.

Reference: page 318

Answer 13.16.   **A, B, and C are correct; D-False**

Wegener's granulomatosis (WG) is a rapidly fatal disease if untreated. A cytotoxic agent (e.g., cyclophosphamide, methotrexate, or azathioprine) should be added to corticosteroids in patients with WG since the latter therapy does not alter the long-term prognosis. Follow-up assessment has revealed a 50% approximate recidivism rate with each of the cytotoxic agents—cytoxan, methotrexate, and azathioprine. There is an approximately 70% infertility rate in women of child-bearing age after treatment for WG with cyclophosphamide; the infertility rate is thought far less following methotrexate or azathioprine therapy.

Reference: page 320

Answer 13.17.   **D**

The male to female ratio is about 2:1 in lymphomatoid granulomatosis (LYG), and most patients are in early middle age. The skin and central nervous system are the two most common extrathoracic sites of involvement. Skin lesions occur in 30–50% of patients. Central nervous system involvement occurs in 30% of patients and is usually manifested by signs and symptoms of a mass lesion. Sinus and upper airway involvement are unusual in LYG. Renal involvement is present in about 45% of patients. Renal involvement in LYG takes the form of a diffuse nodular infiltrate of the renal parenchyma with a characteristic cellular infiltrate, in contrast to the necrotizing glomerulonephritis seen in Wegener's granulomatosis. The pulmonary lesions predominate in the lower lung fields peripherally and are usually bilateral. LYG resembles an indolent lymphoma and may progress to an atypical disseminated lymphoma.

Reference: pages 320–321

Answer 13.18.   A, B, C-True; D, E-False

Allergic angiitis, or Churg-Strauss syndrome, is an eosinophilic granulomatous inflammatory disease with vascular necrosis that frequently involves the pulmonary arteries. Unlike polyarteritis nodosa, it also affects capillaries and venules of the lungs. The disease is primarily seen in patients with an allergic background, often with asthma. Other features include fever, anemia, weight loss, and leukocytosis. The elevation of the erythrocyte sedimentation rate and the degree of peripheral blood eosinophilia are good indicators of disease activity. Allergic angiitis differs from polyarteritis nodosa by its association with an allergic diathesis, its more frequent lung involvement, and the presence of peripheral blood eosinophilia. Corticosteroids have not been shown to significantly increase survival in patients with Churg-Strauss syndrome.

Reference: pages 322–323.

Answer 13.19.   D

Goodpasture's syndrome (antiglomerular basement membrane disease) is one of the pulmonary-renal syndromes characterized by pulmonary hemorrhage. Most patients present with hemoptysis, diffuse alveolar filling on chest films, anemia, and glomerulonephritis. The presence of antiglomerular basement membrane antibodies correlates with disease activity. Anemia is common to all patients and is not hemolytic, but is due to a combination of decreased erythrocyte production and chronic blood loss. Treatment is with combination therapy including corticosteroids, plasmapheresis, and cyclophosphamide or azathioprine. Once renal disease has occurred, it is irreversible, and if renal disease is significant at the time of diagnosis, the prognosis is relatively poor.

Reference: pages 323–325

Answer 13.20.   B, D are correct; A, C are False

There is a male predominance to develop this disease in a ratio of approximately 3.5:1 to 2:1. Early reports on Goodpasture's syndrome indicated a marked male predominance of 9:1, but more recent studies describe lower male to female ratios. Seventy-five percent of patients are between the ages of 17–27 years at the onset of the illness, while the remainder range in age up to 75 years. Urinary findings, which may occur before pulmonary symptoms, include proteinuria, microscopic hematuria, and, less commonly, pyuria. Goodpasture's syndrome demonstrates a predilection for perihilar involvement, while, in contrast to the pulmonary venous congestion and edema of left ventricular failure, Kerley B lines and pleural effusions are not characteristic.

Reference: page 324

Answer 13.21   A, B, C-True; D, E-False

Idiopathic pulmonary hemosiderosis (IPH) is a disease of unknown etiology characterized by repeated episodes of pulmonary hemorrhage, iron-deficiency anemia, and occasionally pulmonary insufficiency. Chest x-ray findings are identical to those of Goodpasture's syndrome. Idiopathic pulmonary hemorrhage may exist without hemoptysis and does not appear to be antibody mediated nor to affect the kidneys. Both diseases may produce an elevated diffusion capacity when recent bleeding is present in the alveoli. With IPH, remission can be permanent, with or without corticosteroid therapy or immunosuppressives, while Goodpasture's syndrome is always fatal without therapy.

Reference: pages 325–326

Answer 13.22. **C**

Pulmonary alveolar proteinosis (PAP) is an alveolar filling process of unknown etiology, manifest by PAS-positive staining, proteinaceous lipid rich material in the alveoli. Treatment in advanced disease requires total lung lavage; other interventions including immunosuppressive therapy have not been shown to be of any benefit. Patients typically demonstrate a restrictive ventilatory impairment on spirometry due to the alveolar filling process. Coexisting infections with nocardia, cryptococcosis, aspergillus, and mucormycosis are common. Mycobacteria are not common infecting organisms. Pneumocystis infection, which may resemble PAP clinically, is ruled out by a negative methenamine silver stain.

Reference: pages 326–328

Answer 13.23. **C, D, E-True; A, B-False**

Toxicity correlates with the total dose of bleomycin given. For total doses administered of more than 300–500 mg, toxicity may approach 50% with an approximate 10% mortality. Older people will have more pulmonary toxicity than younger people. Simultaneous administration of bleomycin and thoracic radiation increases the likelihood of toxicity. Administration of high oxygen concentrations produces synergistic toxicity with bleomycin and a fulminant form of interstitial pneumonitis/fibrosis can develop. Whereas interstitial fibrosis is the usual manifestation of pulmonary toxicity, an apparent corticosteroid responsive hypersensitivity form of toxicity can develop.

Reference: pages 329–331

Answer 13.24. **1-B; 2-A; 3-E; 4-C; 5-D**

Drug induced lung disease is manifest in several forms. Pulmonary fibrosis is common with many cytotoxic and noncytotoxic drugs. Gold salts, penicillamine and sulfasalazine are associated with bronchiolitis obliterans. Penicillamine is the only drug known to cause the pulmonary-renal syndrome. In the chronic setting, nitrofurantoin toxicity may induce blood eosinophilia. Hypersensitivity pneumonitis is closely associated with methotrexate toxicity. Procainamide and hydralazine may induce pleuropulmonary lupus-type reactions.

Reference: pages 330–331

Answer 13.25: **B**

Several drugs are known to induce systemic lupus erythematosus (SLE). Among the more than 20 drugs incriminated are procainamide, hydralazine, diphenylhydantoin, and sulfonamides. Lidocaine is not known to induce SLE.

Reference: page 331

Answer 13.26. **B, D-True; A, C-False**

Amiodarone, a powerful antiarrhythmic, causes lung disease in 4–27% of patients. Pulmonary fibrosis and hypersensitivity pneumonitis or acute pneumonitis can be induced by the drug. The major risk factor is a maintenance dose of more than 400 mg/day. The

DLCO is a highly sensitive predictor of amiodarone toxicity; a DLCO greater than 80% of the pretreatment level virtually excludes amiodarone toxicity. Discontinuation of the drug in conjunction with corticosteroid therapy can reduce the pulmonary disease.

Reference: page 331

Answer 13.27. **A**

Sarcoidosis is a systemic disease usually involving the lungs initially. There is an intense delayed hypersensitivity manifested through T-cells, resulting in noncaseating granuloma formation. Fewer than 10% of patients present with unilateral hilar or isolated paratracheal adenopathy. Patients most often demonstrate a restrictive ventilatory impairment with a reduced DLCO. Bronchoalveolar lavage samples contain predominant lymphocytes of the T-cell variety. ACE levels are elevated in about 60% of active sarcoid patients but are also elevated in Gaucher's disease, leprosy, coccidioidomycosis, osteoarthritis, diabetes mellitus with retinopathy, miliary tuberculosis, primary biliary cirrhosis, atypical mycobacterial infections, inflammatory bowel disease, and some cases of silicosis, asbestosis, and berylliosis.

Reference: pages 332–335

Answer 13.28. **D**

Uveitis, cardiac arrhythmias, neurologic signs—occasionally manifested as palsy of a single cranial nerve (e.g., Bell's palsy), liver dysfunction and hypercalcemia are all complications of sarcoidosis.

Reference: pages 332–337

Answer 13.29. **All are correct**

Skin test anergy to common fungal and tuberculin antigens is a usual feature of active sarcoidosis. There is a paucity of circulating T-lymphocytes among the blood mononuclear cells. Leukopenia occurs in about 30% of patients. The fraction of circulating T-cells is likely to be decreased and the mitogenic response to phytohemagglutinin is reduced in sarcoid patients. B-cells, in contrast, are often increased in acute, active disease.

Reference: page 334

Answer 13.30. **B**

Systemic lupus erythematosus (SLE) is the only disease listed that has not been associated with elevated serum ACE levels. Gaucher's disease, leprosy, coccidioidomycosis, silicosis, asbestosis, berylliosis, and *Mycobacterium intracellulare* infection have been associated with elevated serum ACE levels. Also, osteoarthritis, diabetes mellitus with retinopathy, miliary tuberculosis, primary cirrhosis, and inflammatory bowel disease have all been associated with an elevated serum ACE level. Thus, this test is not pathognomonic of sarcoidosis, although it is likely to be elevated in approximately 60% of patients with active disease.

Reference: page 334

Answer 13.31. **1-D; 2-E; 3-A; 4-C; 5-B**

Moldy redwood dust causes sequoiosis, house dust or bird droppings cause summertime hypersensitivity, moldy cork dust causes suberosis, moldy hay causes Farmer's lung, and moldy sugar cane fiber causes bagassosis.

Reference: page 339

Answer 13.32.   **B**

Hypersensitivity pneumonitis is a relatively common disease and likely underdiagnosed, as the sensitization is usually insidious, and patients may tolerate the mild symptoms until the later stages. Several etiologic agents are known (see Table 13.10 page 339, *Chest Medicine*, 3rd edition). Significant aerosol exposure may result in an immediate asthma-type reaction characterized by air trapping and obstruction with reduction in diffusion capacity. With prolonged exposure in patients prone to continued inflammation, lung destruction occurs, with chest films resembling idiopathic pulmonary fibrosis. Once thought to be uncommon, digital clubbing is now recognized as a significant physical finding in about 50% of patients.

Reference: pages 338–340

Answer 13.33.   **A, B, C-True; D-False**

Total proteins are increased in BAL fluid in patients with chronic hypersensitivity pneumonitis. There are elevated IgG and IgM levels. There is abnormal surfactant composition and large and foamy macrophages have been described. There are high lymphocyte percentages (50–70% of BAL cells).

Reference: pages 339–341

Answer 13.34.   **B, C, D-True; A-False**

Bronchoalveolar fluid from patients with hypersensitivity pneumonitis (HP) generally have high lymphocyte percentages with elevations in immunoglobulin, especially IgG and IgM. Acutely, few patients are studied as the symptoms usually subside; however, the reaction appears to be one of mononuclear cells without eosinophils. Initial treatment in patients with HP should be avoidance of the inciting stimulant. In severe cases, corticosteroids may be indicated, and generally the response is favorable. Skin testing is not routinely incorporated into the diagnostic work-up.

Reference: pages 340–-341

Answer 13.35.   **A, B, C, D-True**

Simple pulmonary eosinophilia is a self limited disease with migratory infiltrates associated with the parasites *Ascaris lumbricoides* and *Strongyloides stercoralis* and the sulfonamide antibiotics. Prolonged pulmonary eosinophilia generally affects women and is associated with occasionally severe systemic symptoms and potential progression to pulmonary fibrosis and honeycombed lung changes. Patients may not have blood eosinophilia. The tropical pulmonary eosinophilia syndrome may mimic attacks of asthma with filarial infection, and the patients appear ill. Large numbers of eosinophils and antibodies to *B. malayi* are found in the BAL fluid. Allergic bronchopulmonary aspergillosis and allergic angiitis with granulomatosis both have pulmonary eosinophilia.

Reference: pages 342–343

Answer 13.36.   **A, C, D-True; B, E-False**

Langerhans's cell granulomatosis (LCG) features proliferation and activation of macrophages often with a form of cell-mediated immunity and a granulomatous tissue reaction. Classically the patients are young males who smoke and present with a pneumothorax and/or chest films noting micronodular densities with interstitial appearing infiltrates that spare the costophrenic angles. A variant of LCG is Hand-Schuller-Christian disease that is a triad of lytic bone lesions, exophthalmus, and pituitary involvement with associated diabetes insipidus. Treatment is controversial, as 10–35% of patients will have spontaneous remissions within several months. Corticosteroids are used, but are not especially effective.

Reference: pages 343–344

chapter 14

Occupational and Environmental Lung Disease

QUESTIONS

Question 14.1. A 37-year-old man presents to a clinic with the complaint of episodic dyspnea. His physical exam is normal, and office spirometry fails to reveal any evidence of restrictive or obstructive lung disease. Chest radiograph is normal. Further history reveals that the dyspneic episodes occur predominantly at night and on weekends. He is employed as an office manager and enjoys woodworking as a hobby. Which one of the following statements is correct in the evaluation of this patient?

A. Bronchoprovocation testing is indicated in the initial work-up of this patient.
B. Failure of these symptoms to improve after avoidance of his woodworking would exclude the diagnosis of occupational asthma.
C. A 20% decrease in the FEV_1 following exposure to the offending agent is diagnostic of occupational asthma.
D. A negative skin test to an antigen in the workplace excludes the compound as the offending agent.

Question 14.2. Match the asthma-inducing agents to the occupations with which they are commonly associated.

A. Acid anhydrides
B. Polyvinyl chloride
C. Diisocyanates (TDI, MDI, HDI)
D. Papain
E. Persulfates

1. Food processors
2. Painters, printers, foam manufacturers
3. Epoxy resin, paint, chemical workers
4. Food wrappers
5. Hairdresser

Question 14.3. A 21-year-old man complains of persistent cough with occasional wheezing. The symptoms developed after exposure to "fumes" while on a weekend military training exercise one month earlier. He is otherwise in good health with a negative past medical history. Which one of the following statements is true regarding the diagnosis of reactive airways dysfunction syndrome (RADS)?

A. RADS may be diagnosed if there is an absence of preceding asthma-like respiratory disease.

B. Patients with RADS will have a negative methacholine or histamine challenge if baseline spirometry is normal.
C. Symptoms associated with RADS usually develop several weeks after the offending episode.
D. Symptoms associated with RADS will disappear after a few days if the patient is not exposed again to the offending agent.

Question 14.4. **True/False statements regarding byssinosis include which of the following?**

A. The risk of developing byssinosis is related to the intensity of dust exposure, duration of exposure and type of fiber
B. Most textile workers who develop the typical byssinosis respiratory symptom complex of chest tightness, cough and wheezing have a history of allergic reactions.
C. During the early stages of byssinosis, symptoms of chest tightness and dyspnea tend to build gradually, with the onset usually noted about 1 hour after the beginning of work.
D. The acute respiratory symptoms of byssinosis are not correlated with a decline in forced expiratory volume in 1-second (FEV_1).

Question 14.5. **True/False statements regarding respiratory effects of grain dust include:**

A. Most grain workers who complain of respiratory symptoms do not have a history of atopy.
B. The combined effects of cigarette smoking and grain on lung function are probably additive.
C. Grain workers who are atopic are at increased risk of developing grain dust asthma.
D. Chronic grain exposure is associated with chronic bronchitis and reduced lung function.

Question 14.6. **A 55-year-old man presents with complaint of chronic cough, with mild dyspnea for 3 days. His is employed as a farmer, and his symptoms developed after shoveling grain from a silo for delivery. He admits to a large exposure to dust at the time. He states that similar symptoms have occurred for years at harvest time, but the symptoms seem to be progressing over the past 5 years with similar exposures. Which one of the following statements is correct in the evaluation of this patient?**

A. Inhalation challenge test with grain dust is likely to produce an immediate but not a delayed reaction.
B. Grain fever may present as hypersensitivity pneumonitis without the chest radiograph findings associated with the disease.
C. Air flow obstruction following both acute and chronic exposure to grain dust is reversible.
D. A history of atopy in grain dust workers predisposes them to development of asthma after exposure.

Question 14.7. **Match the irritant gas to the degree of lethality associated with exposure to it.**

A. Ozone
B. Methyl isocyanate
C. Ammonia
D. Phosgene
E. Oxides of nitrogen (NO, NO_2, N_2O_4)

1. Low
2. Medium
3. High
4. Very high

Question 14.8.   A 30-year-old female complains of dyspnea and burning in her eyes. She states that she was cleaning her swimming pool and adding chlorine to the water. After a few minutes of handling the chlorine, she began to notice the burning sensation and became short of breath. She has no remarkable past medical history. On presentation to the emergency room, the patient is visibly dyspneic and appears ill. Which one of the following statements is correct concerning the initial work-up of this patient?

A. Arterial blood gases, chest radiographs, and bedside spirometry will be abnormal in most patients with inhalational injuries.
B. Highly soluble gases will affect the upper airway prior to the bronchi and alveoli.
C. Lung involvement precedes other systemic signs in cases of inhalation injury.
D. The majority of patients with bronchospasm due to inhalational injuries will not respond to bronchodilator therapy.

Question 14.9.   Match the irritant gas to its description below:

A. Ozone
B. Phosgene
C. Nitrogen dioxide
D. Sulfur dioxide
E. Ammonia

1. Highly water soluble and thus extremely irritating to the mucosa
2. Poorly soluble gas, originally developed for chemical warfare, which penetrates to the distal lung where it causes parenchymal injury
3. Generated during a wide range of industrial operations, including refining of petroleum products and paper manufacturing
4. A highly toxic gas normally found in the atmosphere at very low concentrations, which can be generated by welding; increased amounts are found at high altitude (airplanes) and in urban smog
5. Reddish in color, it is a byproduct of welding, store silage and mining

Question 14.10.   A 41-year-old male fireman is knocked down by a falling beam while involved in putting out a house fire. He is without his mask for several minutes and temporarily loses consciousness. After he is removed from the building he regains consciousness and begins to cough profusely. Upon arrival to the emergency room he is in moderate respiratory distress. An initial arterial oxygen saturation is 92% via pulse oximetry. Which one of the following statements is correct regarding evaluation of this patient?

A. Smoke inhalation victims usually die as a result of inhaling a single chemical asphyxiant.
B. Thermal inhalation injuries are more common than chemical injuries in the average inhalation victim.
C. Permanent sequelae of inhalation injury include interstitial fibrosis and bronchiolitis obliterans.
D. Serial carboxyhemoglobin levels may be useful but are not accurate until 24 hours after the exposure.

Question 14.11.   **Match the metal with its associated health defect.**

A. Metal fume fever
B. Pneumonitis
C. Upper airway irritation
D. Asthma, bronchitis

1. Manganese
2. Osmium
3. Vanadium
4. Chromium

Question 14.12.   **A 60-year-old man worked as a pipefitter for the past 2 years and is concerned about increasing dyspnea with exertion. He has had a normal cardiac work-up and is referred for further evaluation. Chest radiograph reveals hilar lymph nodes with "egg-shell" calcifications. A mediastinoscopy is performed and a lymph node is obtained. Pathology reveals birefringent particles under polarized light. Which one of the following statements is correct regarding these findings?**

A. The physician should consider asbestosis as a likely diagnosis as suggested by the patient's occupation.
B. Without comorbid illness, spirometry uniformly reveals an obstructive ventilatory impairment.
C. Among the connective tissue diseases, rheumatoid arthritis is most commonly associated with silicosis.
D. The prevalence of tuberculosis is greater in patients with this disease than in the average population.

Question 14.13.   **Match the environmental and/or occupational agent to the descriptive statements concerning exposure to it:**

A. Silica
B. Asbestos
C. Beryllium

1. Characteristic chest radiograph shows irregular or linear opacities, which although distributed throughout the lung fields are most prominent in the lower lung zones
2. Calcification of hilar lymph nodes in an "eggshell" pattern may be noted on chest radiograph
3. Causes a chronic pulmonary and systemic granulomatous disease that is similar to sarcoidosis

Question 14.14.   **A 60-year-old man with a history of tobacco use complains of rapidly increasing dyspnea which has developed over the past 2–3 months. He denies any fever, cough, or sputum production. On physical examination, he is generally well developed but has some mild clubbing of his fingers. Further history reveals an occupational history of welding for many years. A chest film demonstrates mild prominence of the pulmonary arteries with "shagginess" of the heart border and some pericardial calcifications. Which one of the following statements is correct in the further evaluation of this patient?**

A. Measurement of the total lung capacity is a sensitive measure of impairment in this patient's condition.
B. Bronchoscopy is usually indicated to diagnose this condition.

C.   Increased lymphocytes, neutrophils, and fibronectin on bronchoalveolar lavage may be associated with reduced lung function in patients with this condition.

D.   High-resolution CT scanning is usually necessary for the diagnosis of this disorder.

Question 14.15.   **Which of the following statements is/are True/False regarding chronic excessive inhalation of coal dust?**

A.   Chronic bronchitis is more common than coal workers' pneumoconiosis (CWP) following excessive inhalation of coal dust.

B.   The small nodular opacities seen on chest radiograph in patients with CWP are due to the presence of coal macules in the lung.

C.   It is unusual to see significant pneumoconiosis in miners who have spent less than 20 years underground.

D.   Coal is less fibrogenic than asbestos or silica.

Question 14.16.   **A 56-year-old coal miner presents with a chest radiograph demonstrating small nodular opacities with some areas of reticular infiltrate. He admits that he coughs for several hours after work each day, and his sputum is occasionally gray to black in color; the cough began to worsen in severity about 6 months ago. He has a 50-pack/year history of tobacco use. Which one of the following statements is correct in the evaluating this patient?**

A.   Centrilobular emphysema seen on his chest radiograph on a chest CI scan may be a result of occupational exposure.

B.   An open lung biopsy is necessary for determining the best course of treatment.

C.   Pulmonary function testing will reveal a specific ventilatory impairment as a result of his occupational exposure.

D.   The presence of serum autoantibodies would exclude a diagnosis of coal worker's pneumoconiosis.

Question 14.17.   **Regarding chronic beryllium disease (CBD), which one of the following statements is true?**

A.   Unlike sarcoidosis, the disease is confined only to the lungs; however, both sarcoidosis and CBD demonstrate noncaseating granulomas.

B.   CBD may represent specific hypersensitivity by a positive lymphocyte transformation test using peripheral blood or BAL lymphocytes.

C.   The disease is apparent after significant exposure to alloys of metals in a few patients after a short duration.

D.   Beryllium is the only environmental cause of granulomatous lung disease.

Question 14.18.   **Choose the agent which is most commonly associated with pulmonary fibrosis following microembolization after intravenous injection of this agent.**

A.   Asbestos
B.   Cobalt
C.   Beryllium
D.   Silica
E.   Talc

Question 14.19.   **Match the following environmental and occupational silicates, dusts, and metals with their respective respiratory tract involvement.**

1.   Talc
2.   Kaolin

3. Graphite
4. Aluminum
5. Nickel
6. Asbestos
7. Chloromethyl ethers

A. A hydrated aluminum silicate that is found in ceramics, paint, paper, and cement
B. Occupational exposures are associated with sinonasal cancers
C. From bauxite, this dust is associated with spontaneous pneumothorax
D. Is associated with small cell carcinomas at an early age
E. The associated lung cancers are located in the lower lobes in two-thirds of cases
F. The dust is a crystallized carbon that may present as a coal worker's pneumoconiosis
G. A hydrated magnesium silicate that can cause idiopathic pulmonary fibrosis; the geologic deposits may contain asbestos

Question 14.20. Which of the following statements are True/False concerning asbestos-related malignancies?

A. Asbestos exposure is associated with an increased incidence primarily of small cell carcinoma of the lung.
B. Asbestos exposure alone is less likely to be associated with carcinoma of the lung than is cigarette smoking alone.
C. The risk for developing malignant mesothelioma is independent of the history of cigarette smoking.
D. Latency between asbestos exposure and lung cancer peaks at 10 years.

Question 14.21. Which of the following exposures is/are causally related to the development of sinonasal cancers?

A. Asbestos
B. Chromium
C. Wood dust
D. Cigarette smoking
E. Nickel

Question 14.22. Which of the following statements regarding asbestos and mesotheliomas is/are correct?

A. Of all cases, 60% are associated with a history of asbestos exposure.
B. The latency period is in the range of 30–40 years.
C. Chrysotile exposure is the asbestos fiber type with the highest potential for inducing mesothelioma.
D. Short, thick asbestos fibers have the highest associated risk for the development of mesothelioma.
E. Mesotheliomas developing in individuals exposed to asbestos do not occur without long-term high level exposure.

ANSWERS

Answer 14.1. **C**

Occupational asthma is the demonstration of variable air flow obstruction or airway hyperresponsiveness associated with an agent or process in the workplace. It is estimated to account for 2–15% of all asthma cases. There is usually a temporal association with a leisure activity (such as woodworking) or an exposure, but the offending agent is not required for the diagnosis. A thorough history and avoidance of stimuli known to cause airway hyperresponsiveness are the initial recommendations. Subsequent diagnostic modalities that may be necessary include bronchoprovocation testing, serial peak flow measurements, and inhalational challenges. Symptoms may persist following prolonged exposure and may develop after years of latency. Negative skin tests are common for low molecular weight compounds (such as diisocyanate) but may be useful for high molecular weight compounds (such as plant proteins).

Reference: pages 361–363

Answer 14.2. **A-3, B-4, C-2, D-1, E-5**

Table 14.2 on page 362 outlines the common occupations associated with asthma-inducing agents.

Reference: page 362

Answer 14.3. **A**

Reactive airways dysfunction syndrome (RADS) is recognized as the presence of symptoms consistent with asthma and nonspecific airway hyperresponsiveness in individuals following a single exposure to an irritating vapor, fire, gas, or smoke. The diagnosis is made by the absence of preceding asthma-like respiratory disease, the onset of symptoms after a single or multiple exposures to a high-level irritant, and onset of symptoms within 24 hours of exposure that persist for at least three months. Spirometry may simulate asthma and methacholine challenge testing may be positive in patients with a normal spirogram. It is important to rule out other asthma-like illnesses in the initial work-up of RADS.

Reference: pages 364–365

Answer 14.4. **A, C-True; B, D-False**

This risk of developing byssinosis is related to the intensity and duration of dust exposure and type of fiber. Most patients who develop the typical respiratory symptom complex have no history of allergic reactions. Symptoms in the early stages of byssinosis develop during the first hour of beginning work. There is a correlation between acute respiratory symptoms of byssinosis and the fall in FEV_1.

Reference: page 365

Answer 14.5. **All are correct**

All four statements are correct. These statements are taken directly from text.

Reference: page 366

Answer 14.6. **B**

Respiratory effects seen with exposure to grain dust are due to the presence of various contaminating materials present, such as fungi, bacteria, mites, insects, animal matter, endotoxins, or agricultural chemicals. Although most grain workers who develop symptoms have a history of atopy, its presence does not place them at increased risk to develop asthma. Grain fever presents similarly to hypersensitivity pneumonitis but without the typical chest radiographic findings. Acute exposures with obstruction are usually reversible; chronic exposure may result in irreversible changes in lung function. Inhalation of grain dust produces both immediate and delayed reactions.

Reference: page 366

Answer 14.7.   A-1, B-3, C-1, D-4, E-3

Ozone, ammonia, acetaldehyde, hydrogen fluoride and hydrogen sulfide all have low lethality when inhaled. Methyl isocyanate and oxides of nitrogen have high lethality upon inhalation, while phosgene gas has a very high lethality when inhaled.

Reference: page 367 (Table 14.3)

Answer 14.8.   B

Inhalation injury results from exposure to different gases, mists, and fumes. These exposures result in inflammation of the upper and lower respiratory tract, depending on the amount and duration of the exposure. Particle size and solubility also determine which part of the respiratory tract is affected; larger and more highly soluble particles affect the upper airways first. Arterial blood gases and chest radiographs are usually normal. If stridor or hoarseness are present, visualization of the vocal cords is indicated and intubation may be necessary if significant edema is present. Bronchospasm usually responds to routine bronchodilator therapy. Permanent impairment presenting as interstitial fibrosis or airway hyperresponsiveness may result in some patients when inflammation persists. Pneumonitis may develop as late as 72 hours after exposure.

Reference: page 367

Answers 14.9.   A-4, B-2, C-5, D-3, E-1

Ammonia is a highly water soluble gas, which is extremely irritable to mucous membranes. *Phosgene,* a poorly soluble gas originally developed for chemical warfare, causes injury to the lung parenchyma. *Sulfur dioxide* is generated from petroleum products and paper manufacturing. *Ozone,* a highly toxic gas normally in the atmosphere at very low concentration, is found in urban smog. *Nitrogen dioxide* is a reddish gas liberated whenever nitrogen containing material is burned.

Reference: page 367

Answer 14.10.   C

The severity of smoke inhalation injuries depends on the magnitude of the exposure and the specific chemical inhaled. Most fires release multiple toxic inhalants including acrolein, hydrogen chloride, and hydrogen cyanide. Thermal injury burns include aerosolized liquids or particles (e.g., metallic oxides), which have a greater heat capacity than dry air. Initial evaluation includes chest auscultation, arterial blood gas analysis with carboxyhemoglobin levels, and assessment for facial or oropharyngeal burns. Permanent sequelae are not common, but when present may include interstitial pulmonary fibrosis, bronchiolitis obliterans, nonspecific airway hyperresponsiveness, and chronic bronchitis.

Reference: pages 368–369

Answer 14.11.   A-1, B-4, C-2, D-3

See Table 14.4 for a summary of the various metal fumes and the conditions associated with exposure to them.

Reference: page 368

Answer 14.12.   **D**

Silicosis is an interstitial fibrosing disease with develops after exposure to dust from mining and quarrying. It may also present after acute or chronic exposure, unlike asbestosis, which is apparent up to 15 years after the exposure. This patient's prior occupation is important, as asbestos exposure from pipe fitting may not be apparent for many years. Scleroderma is the connective tissue disease most often associated with silicosis. Spirometry demonstrates a restrictive impairment unless other factors, such as history of tobacco use, are present which may cause obstructive impairment. *Mycobacterium tuberculosis* as well as atypical mycobacteria are more common in silicosis patients, and often are hard to recognize due to superimposed silicotic disease.

Reference: pages 371–373

Answer 14.13.   **A-2, B-1, C-3**

Asbestos, which occurs in pipe fitters, sheet metal workers, insulation workers, pipe fitters, welders, and asbestos removal workers is associated with opacities in all lung zones but most commonly in the lower lung zones. Although occasionally sarcoidosis causes a pattern of eggshell calcification noted on the chest radiograph, this pattern is classically associated with silicosis, a disease developing in sandblasters, pottery workers, and those working in the manufacture of glass, tiles, and bricks. Beryllium is a chronic pulmonary and systemic granulomatous disease similar to sarcoidosis.

Reference: pages 371–380

Answer 14.14.   **C**

Asbestosis produces a mild leukocytic infiltration of the interstitial spaces, accompanied by varying degrees of organizing fibrosis after inhalation of asbestos fibers. The particles are phagocytized by alveolar macrophages which, when activated, release cytokines and inflammatory mediators. Patients develop a restrictive ventilatory impairment; however, if the patient smokes, the sensitivity of measurement of the total lung capacity is lost. The diagnosis is made by taking a thorough history along with clinical, radiographic, and pulmonary function assessments. The presence of inflammatory cells (e.g., lymphocytes and neutrophils) and fibronectin has been associated with a reduction in lung function. A high-resolution CT scan does not identify changes that are specific for asbestosis.

Reference: pages 373–375

Answer 14.15.   **All are True**

Chronic bronchitis is more common than CWP. Coal macules cause the small nodular opacities in the lungs. Long periods of exposure (20 years or more) are usually required for development of CWP. Both asbestos and silica are more fibrogenic than coal.

Reference: pages 376–377

Answer 14.16.   **A**

Coal worker's pneumoconiosis (CWP) is the presence of coal dust, usually anthracite, in the terminal respiratory units, manifest by reticular nodular opacities on chest films. The opacities are the result of alveolar macrophages phagocytizing the dust particles after many years of exposure. As a result of prolonged oxidant products and macrophage activators, centrilobular emphysema may develop as the parenchyma is destroyed or distorted by the walling-off process. Spirometry may demonstrate restriction, obstruction, or mixed components at any time in the disease. Asbestosis, silicosis, and coal worker's pneumoconiosis are all associated with an increased prevalence of serum autoantibodies. The diagnosis is made based upon the history and duration of exposure, clinical symptoms, and chest films.

Reference: pages 376–377

Answer 14.17. **B**

Chronic beryllium disease (CBD) is a chronic pulmonary and systemic granulomatous disease which is similar to sarcoidosis but is caused by chronic beryllium exposure. Beryllium is present as an alloy in some metals such as copper, aluminum, and nickel. Noncaseating granulomas may be found anywhere in the body and is believed to occur as a disorder of cell mediated immunity including a beryllium specific delayed-type hypersensitivity reaction. The hypersensitivity reaction can be manifest by a positive lymphocyte transformation test. Aluminum and titanium exposure have been reported to induce pulmonary granulomatous reactions.

Reference: pages 377–379

Answer 14.18. **E**

Intravenous drug abusers may inject talc, which embolizes to the lungs and can lead to pulmonary fibrosis.

Reference: page 380

Answer 14.19. **1-G; 2-A; 3-F; 4-C; 5-B; 6-E; 7-D**

Talc is a hydrated magnesium silicate known to cause IPF in some patients, and when used for procedures like pleurodesis, it must be asbestosis free as often fibers will be present in talc. Kaolin is a hydrated aluminum silicate found in many products including ceramics, paint, paper, and cement. Graphite is crystallized carbon that may present as small to large nodular densities on chest film much like coal worker's pneumoconiosis. Aluminum dust exposure is associated with a spontaneous pneumothorax in those who develop interstitial lung disease. Sinonasal cancers are associated with nickel as well as chromium, cutting oils, formaldehyde, and wood smoke. Lung cancers are associated with asbestosis exposure after many years, especially in smokers, and the nodules are present in the lower lobes in two-thirds of patients, although this is a nonspecific finding. Chloromethyl ether exposures are associated with small cell carcinomas at an early age.

Reference: pages 380–385

Answer 14.20. **B, C-True; A, D-False**

All major cell types of lung cancer are associated with asbestos exposure. Asbestos exposure alone, without cigarette smoking, presents a minimally increased risk of developing lung cancer over non-smoking individuals who are not exposed to asbestos. However, in an asbestos exposed worker who smokes cigarettes the incidence of lung cancer is markedly increased over non-smokers and non-smoking asbestos workers. Cigarette smoking is not causally related to the development of mesothelioma. Latency between asbestos exposure and development of lung cancer peaks at 20–30 years.

Reference: pages 384, 396

Answer 14.21.   **B, C and E are correct**

Although asbestos, cigarette smoking, and alcohol are not associated with an increased incidence of sinonasal cancer, nickel, wood dust, chromium, cutting oils, formaldehyde, and wood dust are associated causally with sinonasal cancer.

Reference: page 386

Answer 14.22.   **B**

At least 80% of cases of mesothelioma are associated with a history of asbestos exposure. The latency period is in the range of 30–40 years. Chrysotile is the asbestos fiber type least likely to cause mesothelioma, while the amphiboles, crocidolite and amosite, appear to have the highest potential. Long, thin, not short, thick fibers have the highest associated risk for the development of mesothelioma. Even short-term, low-level exposure has been associated with development of mesothelioma.

Reference: page 386

chapter 15

Lung Neoplasms

QUESTIONS

Question 15.1. **True/False statements regarding the prevalence and incidence of lung cancer include:**

A. Lung cancer is the most common malignant neoplasm in men throughout the world.
B. The mortality from lung cancer and stomach cancer has been rising in men and women over the past four decades.
C. Ten percent of patients with lung cancer are under 40 years of age
D. Between 1953 and 1983 lung cancer deaths increased in both men and women but more in men.
E. Breast cancer is the leading cause of death in women followed by lung cancer.

Question 15.2. **True/False statements regarding the risk of developing lung cancer include:**

A. After correlation for smoking, a high dietary intake of carotene (pro-Vitamin A) is associated with a lower incidence of lung cancer than a low dietary intake of carotene.
B. Cigarette smokers exposed in their occupation to large amounts of silica have an increased risk of developing lung cancer.
C. Passive smoking increases the incidence of lung cancer.
D. Cigarette smoking adds significantly to the propensity of brake liners and pipe fitters to develop asbestos-induced lung cancer.
E. Genetic factors predispose to lung cancer.

Question 15.3. **The risk of developing lung cancer is directly related to total exposure to cigarette smoke as measured by (answer True/False):**

A. The depth of inhalations
B. The levels of tar and nicotine in the cigarettes smoked
C. The duration of smoking in years
D. The age of initiation of smoking
E. The number of cigarettes smoked

Question 15.4. **Which of the following statements regarding the etiology of lung cancer are true/false?**

A. Mortality is higher in rural than in urban regions.
B. In non-smokers, the predominant lung cancer cell type is squamous cell carcinoma.
C. An average lifetime of passive smoke exposure to a smoking spouse increases a nonsmoker's low risk by about 35% compared with the risk of 1000% for a lifetime of active smoking.

D. In contrast to white women, in whom new lung cancer cases have dropped recently, lung cancer in white males is still increasing.

E. Uranium exposure is strongly associated with carcinoma of the lung, particularly small cell carcinoma.

Question 15.5.   Choose the most common lung cancer cell type.

A. Adenocarcinoma
B. Large cell carcinoma
C. Alveolar cell carcinoma
D. Small cell carcinoma
E. Squamous cell carcinoma

Question 15.6.   Bronchoalveolar cell carcinoma (alveolar cell carcinoma) is considered a subtype of which lung cancer cell type?

A. Squamous cell carcinoma
B. Adenocarcinoma
C. Adenosquamous cell
D. Large cell carcinoma
E. Small cell carcinoma

Question 15.7.   Match the lung cancer cell type most closely associated with the following descriptions.

A. Adenocarcinoma
B. Squamous cell carcinoma
C. Alveolar cell carcinoma
D. Small cell carcinoma
E. Giant cell variant of large cell carcinoma

1. In about two-thirds of cases, this tumor presents as a proximal or hilar lesion; it is uncommon for this tumor to metastasize early.
2. This tumor is often multicentric or lobar in location.
3. Of these tumors, 55–60% are located in the periphery, and the brain and bone are frequent sites of metastases.
4. Of these tumors, 75–80% present as proximal lesions and the tumor is usually extensive, often with distant metastases.
5. This highly aggressive tumor has a predilection for metastasis to the intestines.

Question 15.8.   Select the lung cancer cell type most commonly associated with hypercalcemia.

A. Small cell carcinoma
B. Squamous cell carcinoma
C. Adenocarcinoma
D. Large cell carcinoma
E. Alveolar cell carcinoma

Question 15.9.   Choose the *incorrect* statement among the following statements regarding patients with lung cancer and hypertrophic osteoarthropathy (HOA).

A. Its occurrence is distributed equally among squamous cell, adenocarcinoma and large cell carcinoma lung cancer cell types.

B. Although the mechanism of development of the tissue changes is unknown, an increase in blood flow in the affected portions of the limbs has been described and reverts following successful treatment of the underlying condition.

C. Removal of the pulmonary lesion induces a dramatic remission of arthralgia.
D. It occurs most frequently in small cell lung tumors.
E. In addition to lung cancer, HOA occurs in patients with cystic fibrosis.

Question 15.10. **Which one of the following statements is *not* true regarding the chest radiograph in lung neoplasms?**

A. Most lung cancers are detected by the standard chest radiograph.
B. Lesions less than 0.5 to 6 mm in diameter are unlikely to be detected.
C. Small cell lung cancer is the lung cancer cell type that cavitates most frequently.
D. Spiculation of lung lesions is more indicative of malignancy than a smooth border.
E. A bronchogenic carcinoma may have eccentric calcification.

Question 15.11. **Select the best imaging technique for assessing superior sulcus lesions.**

A. High resolution computed tomography (HRCT)
B. Magnetic resonance imaging (MRI)
C. Plain chest radiograph
D. Conventional tomography
E. Chest CT with contrast

Question 15.12. **A 51-year-old secretary presents for a check-up. She has recently moved to your area to assume a new position. She has a 50 pack/year history of cigarette smoking and has always been healthy at annual check-ups.**

Her physician examination and routine laboratory studies are normal. However, a routine posteroanterior (PA) and lateral chest radiograph shows a 2.4 cm × 2.9 cm smooth, well-demarcated lesion in the lateral basal subsegment of the left lower lobe.

The appropriate initial step for the patient's physician would be to:

A. Order a transthoracic needle biopsy
B. Order a chest CT scan
C. Obtain cone-down conventional tomograms of the lesion to learn if it is calcified
D. Obtain prior chest radiographs from former physician(s)
E. Ask a pulmonologist to perform bronchoscopy

Question 15.13. **Which of the following statements is/are TRUE/FALSE regarding solitary pulmonary nodules?**

A. A sharply defined smooth margin rules out malignancy.
B. Diffuse, central, or laminated calcification of the lesion renders benignity highly likely.
C. Stability of the nodule (not growing for at least 1 year) is a generally accepted criteria for benignity.
D. Calcification of a lung lesion is most accurately determined from magnetic resonance imaging.
E. Stippled, eccentric calcification patterns rule out malignancy.

Questions 15.14–15.16. **A 72-year-old retired male asbestos worker with a 100 pack/year history of cigarette smoking presents with a 4 to 5 cm cavitary squamous cell carcinoma invading the chest wall. Chest CT scan shows no other lung lesions and the mediastinum and hila are normal. A head CT is negative. Bone scan shows only increased uptake in the area where the lesion invades the chest wall.**

Choose the simple best answer in each of the following questions regarding this patient.

15.14. **At what stage is this tumor?**

A. Stage IV
B. Stage IIIB
C. Stage I
D. Stage IIIA
E. Stage II

15.15. **What is the appropriate TNM classification of this lesion?**

A. T1N2M0
B. T2N1M0
C. T4N0M0
D. T3N0M1
E. T3N0M0

15.16. **What is the appropriate therapy for this lesion?**

A. Radiation therapy
B. Brachytherapy
C. Chemotherapy
D. Surgical resection
E. Laser therapy

Question 15.17. **Match the clinical stage grouping with the description.**

A. Stage I
B. Stage II
C. Stage IIIa
D. Stage IIIb
E. Stage IV

1. A 63-year-old man with a 4-cm large cell carcinoma of the right upper lobe and left supraclavicular lymph node involvement
2. A 79-year-old woman with a 5-cm squamous cell carcinoma in the periphery of the lingula and a tumor positive ipsilateral hilar lymph node without mediastinal or extra thoracic involvement
3. An 89-year-old man with a 15-cm large cell carcinoma in the right lower lobe, no hilar or mediastinal positive lymph nodes, and no distant metastasis
4. A 39-year-old man with a central proximal left main stem bronchus squamous cell carcinoma invading the esophagus without distant metastasis
5. A 62-year-old woman with atherosclerotic heart disease, a right upper lobe 2-cm peripheral adenocarcinoma, and a transudative left pleural effusion with negative cytology at thoracentesis and biopsy negative pleura at thoracoscopy; there is no nodal involvement or distant metastasis.

Question 15.18. **For each patient with non-small cell lung cancer described below, select the most appropriate staging classification (A-E).**

A. Stage I
B. Stage II
C. Stage IIIA
D. Stage IIIB
E. Stage IV

1. A patient with a 4.8 cm widest-diameter large cell carcinoma in the middle lobe, with one ipsilateral hilar lymph node containing tumor and tumor involvement in one ipsilateral mediastinal lymph node.

2. A patient with a squamous cell carcinoma in the mid trachea invading posteriorly into the lumen of the esophagus with negative hilar and mediastinal lymph nodes and no other evidence of disease.
3. A patient with squamous cell carcinoma of the proximal left main stem bronchus invading the carina, and with no other evidence of disease.
4. A patient with a 6-cm widest-diameter adenocarcinoma in the periphery of the middle lobe with no hilar or mediastinal adenopathy or evidence of other disease.

Question 15.19. **Match the primary tumor (T) status to the description.**

A. T0
B. T1
C. T2
D. T3
E. T4

1. A squamous cell carcinoma originating at the entrance of the right upper lobe and extending proximally with invasion through the right lateral tracheal wall 3 cm above the carina
2. An endobronchial squamous cell tumor 2 cm in widest diameter situated 0.5 cm above the entrance to the left lower lobe carcinoma without distal atelectasis
3. A 2.8 cm adenocarcinoma invading the visceral pleural
4. A large cell carcinoma of the left lower lobe extending into the adjacent diaphragm
5. A central left lung adenosquamous cell carcinoma extending into the pericardium without involving the heart

Question 15.20. **Which of the following questions regarding TNM subsets of non-small cell lung cancer is/are TRUE/FALSE?**

A. Invasion of a vertebral body is a T4 lesion
B. Tumor metastasis to an ipsilateral supraclavicular lymph node is labeled N2
C. A non-small cell tumor located within 1 cm of the main carcinoma not involving the carina is a T3 lesion
D. A tumor invading the aorta is a T3 lesion

Question 15.21. **Which of the following statements regarding surgery for non-small cell lung cancer is/are TRUE/FALSE?**

A. Patients with chest wall involvement of tumor (T3N0M0) have an 18% 5-year survival after resection.
B. Stage I patients with adenocarcinomas have a better prognosis than Stage I patients with squamous cell carcinoma
C. Patients with Stage I non-small lung cancers greater than 3 cm have a lower 5-year survival than patients with tumors equal to or less than 3 cm.
D. The 5-year survival for postsurgical Stage II (T1N1M0 or T2N1M0) tumors following resection is about 40–50%.

Question 15.22. **Which of the following statements regarding radiation therapy for small cell and non-small cell lung cancers is/are TRUE/FALSE?**

A. Cranial irradiation reduces the development of metastases and improves survival in patients with small cell lung cancer.
B. Small cell carcinomas are radiosensitive.
C. Radiation therapy of patients with small peripheral Stage I (T1N0M0) non-small cell carcinomas and medical contraindications to surgical resection does not enhance 5-year survival.

D. Large cell undifferentiated tumors respond least favorably of the primary lung cancer cell types to radiation therapy.

Question 15.23. **For the patients with lung cancer described below, select the therapy of choice:**

A. Chemotherapy
B. Laser therapy
C. Radiation therapy
D. Surgical resection
E. Chemotherapy and radiation therapy

1. A 59-year-old man with a forced expiratory volume in one-second (FEV_1) of 1.8 liters and normal cardiac function with a left endobronchial squamous cell carcinoma within 2 cm of the carina but not involving the carina. Physical examination and laboratory tests (complete blood count, liver and renal function tests, calcium, phosphorus and electrolytes) are all normal. There is no mediastinal or hilar disease on chest CT scan and a quantitative ventilation/perfusion lung scan indicates that the right lung contributes 55% of perfusion and ventilation, whereas the left lung contributed 45%, and the postoperative predicted FEV_1 is 65% predicted, 990 ml.
2. A 49-year-old man with a peripheral left upper lobe small cell carcinoma and metastases to the parietal lobe of the brain.
3. A 54-year-old woman with normal lung function and a small cell lung cancer of the right upper lobe with a biopsy-proven tumor positive right supraclavicular lymph node.

Question 15.24. **The following questions are True/False regarding carcinoid tumor (bronchial adenoma).**

A. 70% present as peripheral lesions.
B. These tumors occur slightly more frequently in men.
C. Hemoptysis is rare in patients with this lesion.
D. Most patients are diagnosed in their 60s.
E. Operative removal is indicated.

Question 15.25. **The following statements are True/False regarding hamartoma.**

A. Characteristically the lesion is round and has sharply defined margins.
B. This tumor is well encapsulated.
C. Calcification is evident on chest radiograph in 50% of cases.
D. This is the most common benign lung tumor.
E. The majority of these lesions arise within a major or segmental bronchus.

ANSWERS

Answer 15.1. **A - True; B, C, D, E - False**

Lung cancer is the most common malignant neoplasm in men throughout the world. Although lung cancer death rates have been rising, mortality from stomach cancer has decreased over the past several decades (Figs. 15.1 and 15.2). Less than 5% of patients with lung cancer are under 40 years of age. A staggering 360% increase in lung cancer deaths occurred in women between 1953 and 1983, contrasted with a 184% increase in men. Recently, lung cancer surpassed breast cancer as the leading cancer killer in women.

Reference: pages 393 and 394

Answer 15.2. **A, C, D, E - True; B - False**

Persons whose diet contains large amounts of carotene (pro-vitamin A), when corrected for cigarette smoking, seem to have a significantly lower incidence of lung cancer than persons who have a low dietary pro-vitamin A intake, although this is currently under wide investigation in prospective trials. There are not definitive data that silica exposure increases the incidence of lung cancer. Apparently there is an increased incidence of lung cancer in persons who do not smoke cigarettes but who are widely exposed to passive smoking, particularly non-smoking spouses of heavy cigarette smokers. Asbestos exposure combined with cigarette smoking substantially increases the incidence of lung cancer over that of persons not exposed to asbestos and who do not smoke cigarettes. Cigarette smoking, though, is *the* major factor in asbestos-associated lung cancer. Genetic factors clearly predispose lung cancer; however, the specific, important genetic factors are still being elucidated.

Reference: pages 394–398

Answers 15.3. **A, B, C, D, E - True**

All five statements regarding smoking and lung cancer are true.

Reference: page 394

Answer 15.4. **C, E - True; A, B, D - False**

Mortality from lung cancer is higher in urban areas than in rural regions, suggesting an etiologic role for air pollutants. Adenocarcinoma is the predominant lung cancer cell type in non-smokers. Passive smoking appears to increase the incidence of lung cancer in non-smokers, but much less than active smoking. Lung cancer has decreased in white males but continues to increase in women. Small cell lung cancer has been especially implicated in individuals exposed to uranium.

Reference: pages 395 and 396

Answer 15.5. **A**

Over the past few decades adenocarcinoma (33–35%) has surpassed squamous cell carcinoma (30–32%) as the most common lung cancer cell type. Large cell carcinoma comprises 15–18% and small cell carcinoma 20–25% of all lung carcinomas. Alveolar cell carcinoma accounts for 2–4% of all lung carcinomas.

Reference: page 398

Answer 15.6. **B**

Bronchoalveolar carcinomas (so-called alveolar cell carcinomas) are considered adenocarcinomas. As a group, they comprise at least 2–4% of all lung carcinomas.

Reference: page 398

Answer 15.7. **1-B; 2-C; 3-A, 4-D; 5-E**

Both squamous cell and small cell lung cancers are predominantly central lesions, but the latter, unlike the former, tends to metastasize to distant sites early. Adenocarcinoma, frequently a peripheral tumor, has a predilection for brain and bone metastases. Bronchioloalveolar carcinoma (alveolar cell carcinoma) is often multicentric or lobar in location. Giant cell variant of large cell carcinoma has an unexplained propensity to metastasize to the intestines.

Reference: pages 399–401

Answer 15.8.   **B**

Squamous cell carcinoma is the predominant lung cancer cell type associated with hypercalcemia.

Reference: page 404

Answer 15.9.   **D**

All the statements are correct, except HOA rarely, if ever, occurs in patients with small cell lung cancer.

Reference: page 405

Answer 15.10.   **C**

Squamous cell carcinoma is the lung cancer cell type that most frequently cavitates. Small cell carcinoma rarely, if ever, cavitates.

Reference: page 406

Answer 15.11.   **B**

MRI is the best technique for assessing superior sulcus lesions, for it can most clearly distinguish the extent of invasion, including potential brachial plexus involvement.

Reference: page 410

Answer 15.12.   **D**

When a lung lesion is identified in a patient, the first step is to obtain prior chest radiographs. If the lesion on chest radiograph has been stable for two or more years without evidence of growth, the lesion is likely benign and can continue to be watched. Other listed options in this situation would be considered only after it had been established by reviewing previous chest radiographs that the lesion had grown or is new within two years. Obtaining a prior chest radiograph(s) might avoid a costly work-up. If no previous chest radiographs are available, a chest CT scan with contrast should be done to identify other lung lesions and to ascertain whether there is evidence of hilar or mediastinal lymph node involvement. A bronchoscopy is also indicated if the lung lesion is new, to determine the extent of any endobronchial involvement or the presence of unexpected occult endobronchial lung lesions, and to try to diagnose the cause of the lung lesion through forceps and brush biopsy, as well as lavage or washing. Cone-down tomograms are rarely used because the chest CT scan is more sensitive for assessing lung lesions.

Reference: pages 406, 407, 410–441

Answers 15.13.   **B - True; A, C, D, E - False**

Spiculation on poorly defined smooth margins of lesions suggests a malignancy whereas a sharply defined smooth margin does not rule out a malignancy. If calcification is present in a diffuse, central, laminated or "popcorn pattern," benignity of the solitary pulmonary nodule is highly likely. Stippled, eccentric calcification patterns do not rule out malignancy. Visible calcification can often by determined from standard tomograms or from thin-section, high-resolution CT (HRCT). To detect and quantify calcification in solitary pulmonary nodules, CT densitometry can be employed, particularly if there is no visual evidence of calcification in the lesion. The use of a reference phantom may be required with densitometry to calibrate the CT scanner. Magnetic resonance imaging is not used to detect tissue calcification. The establishment from review of prior chest radiographs that the solitary nodule has been stable (not growing) for at least 2 years, not 1 year, is a generally accepted criteria for benignity.

Reference: page 412

Answer 15.14. **D**

Answer 15.15. **E**

Answer 15.16. **D**

This non-small cell cancer invades the chest wall and therefore is a clinical T3N0M0 lesion, Stage IIIA. Surgery should provide approximately a 35% 5-year survival.

Reference: pages 408 and 413

Answer 15.17. **1-D; 2-B; 3-A; 4-D; 5-A**

The patient with large cell carcinoma and supraclavicular lymph node involvement is at Stage IIIb (T2N3M0). Supraclavicular lymph node metastasis is N3. The woman with the tumor positive ipsilateral hilar lymph node (N1) is at Stage II (T2N1M0). Although the tumor is huge 15 cm (T2) in the 89-year-old man, without nodal involvement or distant metastasis, this is a Stage I lesion. Obviously, the prognosis is worse in large Stage I vs. small Stage I lesions. Esophageal invasion (T4) renders the 39-year-old man with a central squamous cell carcinoma at Stage IIIb. Clearly, not all pleural effusions in patients with lung cancer are due to spread of tumor (T4). This effusion may have been due to congestive heart failure. This tumor is at Stage I (T1N0M0).

Reference: page 408

Answer 15.18. **1-C; 2-D; 3-D; 4-A**

The revised American Joint Committee Staging Classification is the basis for decisions regarding therapy and prognosis for patients with non-small cell lung cancer. For example, patients with Stage I or II non-small carcinoma of the lung are candidates for surgical extirpation of the primary tumor as long as their cardiovascular and pulmonary status is adequate. Selected patients with Stage IIIA disease are candidates for surgical removal of the lung carcinoma with intent to cure, while patients with Stage IIIB or IV disease are not candidates for surgical resection.

The patient with a 4.8-cm widest-diameter large cell carcinoma in the middle lobe with involvement of one ipsilateral hilar lymph node and one ipsilateral mediastinal lymph node without presence of distant disease has a Stage IIIA (T2N2M0) tumor. If there were no mediastinal involvement, this patient would have been at Stage II (T2N1M0). The 5-year survival of clinical Stage II disease is about 35% compared with a 5-year survival of 20% or less in patients with clinical Stage IIIA disease. If cardiovascular and pulmonary status are acceptable, patients at Stage II and some patients at Stage IIIA are candidates for surgical excision with intent to cure. Frequently, a pneumonectomy is required to remove all tumor in patients with hilar lymph node involvement.

The patient with squamous cell carcinoma of the trachea invading posteriorly through the wall into the lumen of the esophagus has a Stage IIIB lesion (T4N0M0). Whenever another thoracic visceral organ is involved with a non-small cell carcinoma of the lung, the lesion is considered unresectable for cure and in advanced stage. Thus, for example, patients with tumor involvement of the esophagus, the heart, and major blood vessels are classified as T4. Therapy for these patients is likely to be palliative in intent.

The patient with squamous cell carcinoma of the proximal left main stem bronchus invading the carina has Stage IIIB disease (T4N0M0) and because the tumor invades the carina would in most cases not be considered a surgical candidate. Rarely, a plastic procedure can be accomplished on such patients, placing a graft in place of the carina. However, in most such patients the tumor involvement in the area of the carina is too extensive to permit such radical surgery. This patient would likely receive palliative external beam irradiation or laser therapy with or without brachytherapy. If the tumor had been within 2 cm of the main carina but not involving it (Stage IIIA, T3N0M0), surgical removal likely would have been possible.

Even though the last (fourth) patient has a large tumor (6-cm widest diameter), this lesion is in the periphery of the lung and is not associated with adenopathy or distant disease. Accordingly, this is a clinical Stage I lesion (T2N0M0) with a substantially lower 5-year patient survival (about 50%) following surgical resection than a similar clinical Stage I peripheral lesion with a much smaller widest diameter (for example, a less than 3-cm T1N0M0 lesion—about 70–75% 5-year patient survival after surgical resection).

Reference: pages 408, 409, 413, and 414

Answer 15.19.   **1-E; 2-B; 3-C; 4-D; 5-D**

A non-small cell tumor invading the trachea is T4. A 2 cm distal endobronchial non-small cell tumor without distal atelectasis is T1. A 2.8 cm non-small cell tumor invading the visceral pleura only is a T2 lesion. Non-small cell lung cancer with diaphragm or pericardial (without heart) extension is a T3 lesion.

Reference: page 408

Answer 15.20.   **A, C - True; B, D - False**

Tumors invading of a vertebral body, great vessels, heart, trachea and esophagus are T4 lesions. A lesion within 2 cm of the carina but not involving it is a T3 lesion. Tumor metastasis to a supraclavicular lymph node is an N3 lesion.

Reference: page 408 (Table 15.6)

Answer 15.21.   **D - True; A, B, C - False**

The 5-year survival of patients with T3N0M0 tumors with chest wall invasion is approximately 35–40%. Most studies suggest patients with squamous cell carcinomas have a better 5-year survival than those with adenocarcinoma. Postsurgical Stage II tumors have a 40% (T2N1M0) to 52 or 54% (T1N1M0) 5-year patient survival (Table 15.8, p. 413). The larger the Stage I non-small cell tumor the worse the prognosis.

Reference: page 413 (Table 15.8)

Answer 15.22.   **B, D - True; A, C - False**

Although cranial irradiation decreases CNS metastases in small cell lung cancer, survival is not altered. Small cell carcinomas are radiosensitive. In patients with small Stage I (T1N0M0) peripheral non-small cell tumors, continuous cycle radiation therapy may achieve between a 25 and 50% 5-year survival. Large cell carcinomas are the least radiosensitive of the primary lung cancers.

Reference: page 414

Answer 15.23.   **1-D; 2-E; 3-A**

The man in item 1 has Stage IIIA non-small cell carcinoma, which is within 2 cm of the carina but not involving it (T3). This patient is a potential candidate for surgical resection with approximately a 15%–20% 5-year survival if surgical staging shows the tumor does not involve the main carina or at surgery there are no tumor-positive mediastinal or hilar lymph nodes. Likely, the patient will require a left pneumonectomy, and should tolerate this procedure because the predicted postoperative FEV_1 is greater than 60% predicted and greater than 800 ml, namely 990 ml. This postoperative FEV_1 is predicted on the basis of the preoperative FEV_1 of 1800 ml and 55% perfusion determined by quantitative ventilation/perfusion lung scan in the right lung which will remain in place after the left pneumonectomy. The 990 ml residual FEV_1 is 55% of 1800 ml.

The woman in case 2 has advanced small cell carcinoma of the lung with metastasis to the brain. Although the primary therapy for small cell carcinoma of the lung is chemotherapy, in patients with small cell or non-small cell carcinoma of the lung with established metastasis to the brain, it is appropriate to irradiate the head. Similarly, if there is metastasis to the skeleton which is painful or which puts the patient at risk for pathologic fracture (for example, greater trochanter of the femur), radiation therapy is indicated. This patient should receive both systemic chemotherapy and local radiation to the head.

In patients with either non-small cell or small cell tumors, such as the patient in item 3, supraclavicular lymph node metastasis indicates unresectability for cure. As stated, the primary therapy for small cell lung cancer is chemotherapy. In the United States some centers add radiation therapy, in addition to chemotherapy, particularly when the disease in the thorax has been well controlled with chemotherapy.

Reference: pages 408, 409, 413, 415

Answer 15.24.   **E - True; A, B, C, D - False**

Of carcinoid tumors, 90% are located in a major or segmental bronchus. These lesions are slightly more common in women. Hemoptysis occurs in one-third of patients. Most patients are diagnosed in their thirties and have had symptoms for over 5 years when the tumor is first diagnosed. To prevent severe hemoptysis and distal infection, surgical removal is indicated.

Reference: page 416

Answer 15.25.   **A, D - True; B, C, E - False**

Hamartoma is characteristically round and has sharply defined margins. No capsule is present. Calcification is seen on chest radiograph in 10% and usually appears as small flecks throughout the lesion. This is the most common benign lung tumor. Only 8–20% of the lesions arise within a major or segmental bronchus.

Reference: page 417

chapter 16

Respiratory Tract Infections

QUESTIONS

Question 16.1. **Which of the following statements are TRUE or FALSE concerning the epidemiology of pneumonia?**

A. There are an estimated one million cases of community-acquired pneumonia requiring hospitalization annually in the United States.
B. Pneumonia is the sixth leading cause of death in the United States.
C. Nosocomial pneumonias carry the highest mortality of any nosocomial infections.
D. The majority of nosocomial pneumonias are bacterial in origin.

Question 16.2. **Which of the following groups is/are at increased risk for infection with *Mycobacterium tuberculosis*?**

A. African Americans
B. Hispanics
C. Asian immigrants
D. Nursing home residents

Question 16.3. **Which of the following respiratory tract sites is/are considered to be sterile in normal individuals?**

A. Alveoli
B. Trachea
C. Nasopharynx
D. Paranasal sinuses

Question 16.4. **Which of the following statements is/are correct regarding the common cold?**

A. There are more than 200 different agents which can cause symptoms of the common cold.
B. Parainfluenza virus is the most common agent causing the common cold.
C. There is an increased risk of developing colds in smokers.
D. Vitamin C has been shown to be useful in decreasing the symptoms and duration of the common cold.

Question 16.5. **Which of the following organisms is LEAST likely to cause sinusitis in a normal immunocompetent host?**

A. *Staphylococcus aureus*
B. *Haemophilus influenzae*
C. *Streptococcus pneumoniae*
D. Rhinovirus

Question 16.6. **Which of the following statements is/are correct regarding acute epiglottitis?**

A. The disease, although more dangerous in infants than children, is actually more common in the adult population.
B. The most common etiologic agent is the parainfluenza virus.
C. Diagnosis is most commonly made by recognition of signs and symptoms as well as radiographic findings; actual examination with tongue blade should not be attempted.
D. The first and most important step in the management of epiglottitis is maintenance of a patent airway.

Question 16.7. **Treatment of pharyngitis caused by** *Streptococcus pneumoniae* **provides all of the following benefits EXCEPT:**

A. Reduction of illness duration
B. Prevention of spread to others
C. Prevention of suppurative complications
D. Prevention of glomerulonephritis

Question 16.8. **The cardinal features of an exacerbation of chronic bronchitis include all of the following EXCEPT:**

A. Dyspnea
B. Fever
C. Increase in sputum purulence
D. Increase in sputum production

Question 16.9. **Determine whether the following statements are TRUE or FALSE regarding acute respiratory infections due to the influenza virus:**

A. Disease due to type B is usually more severe.
B. The presence of antigenic drift and decreasing immunity makes the disease a threat each year, regardless of previous exposure or vaccination.
C. Epidemics usually occur in the late fall and extend into early spring.
D. Influenza A may coexist with other viral infections.
E. When dealing with influenza epidemics in a closed environment (e.g., nursing homes), vaccination should be given to nonimmunized patients and antiviral therapy with rimantadine should be given for 3 days after vaccination.

Question 16.10. **The major route of acquisition for most forms of pneumonia in non-hospitalized patients is:**

A. Inhalation from ambient air
B. Hematogenous spread
C. Direct inoculation from contiguous infected sites
D. Aspiration from a previously colonized upper airway

Question 16.11. **Which of the following processes are involved in the colonization of the lower airways by Gram-negative bacteria?**

A. Decreased mucociliary clearance.
B. Increased tracheal cell capacity to bind bacteria.
C. Decrease in the normal flora of the lower airways that normally inhibits growth of pathogens.
D. Endotracheal intubation.

Question 16.12. **Match each organism listed below with the clinical setting in which it is most likely to be the causative agent of pneumonia:**

A. *Klebsiella pneumoniae*
B. *Haemophilus influenzae*
C. *Pseudomonas aeruginosa*
D. *Streptococcus pneumoniae*
E. *Aspergillus fumigatus*

1. 65-year-old male smoker with chronic bronchitis
2. 20-year-old woman with cystic fibrosis
3. 32-year-old man with leukemia
4. 45-year-old man with chronic alcohol abuse
5. 23-year-old woman with sickle cell anemia and splenectomy

Question 16.13. The most common bacterial pathogen for community-acquired pneumonia for all types of patients is:

A. *Haemophilus influenzae*
B. *Klebsiella pneumoniae*
C. *Moraxella catarrhalis*
D. *Streptococcus pneumoniae*

Question 16.14. Which of the following statements is/are correct regarding pneumonia due to *Streptococcus pneumoniae?*

A. There are 84 different serotypes of pneumococcus, but most infections are caused by one of 23 serotypes.
B. The presence of bacteremia during pneumococcal pneumonia is associated with a greater increase in mortality in patients with AIDS than in the general population.
C. In AIDS patients with pneumococcal pneumonia, bacteremia is more common than in healthy populations of the same age.
D. Infection with pneumococcus is most common in the late fall and early winter.

Question 16.15. Which of the following statements is/are correct concerning pneumonia caused by *Legionella* species?

A. Infection is caused by inhalation of an infected aerosol from a contaminated water source or by aspiration from a colonized oropharynx.
B. The use of corticosteroids is the most significant risk factor for developing nosocomial pneumonia due to *Legionella*.
C. For serologic diagnosis, the urinary antigen test shows high sensitivity and specificity for detecting all serotypes of *Legionella*.
D. Erythromycin is the drug of choice for treating *Legionella* pneumonia.

Question 16.16. Determine whether the following statements are TRUE or FALSE regarding pneumonia secondary to aspiration.

A. Aspiration pneumonias are more commonly seen on the left side.
B. When aspiration occurs outside the hospital, as in patients with seizures or stroke, the most common bacteria causing pneumonia are anaerobes that have colonized the oropharynx.
C. Treatment of nosocomial aspiration is with penicillin G and/or clindamycin.
D. Corticosteroids and prophylactic antibiotics have been shown to be of benefit in preventing pneumonia after witnessed aspiration.

Question 16.17. Match the characteristics of the atypical pneumonias listed below with the organisms which are most likely responsible:

A. Bloody pleural effusion
B. Mental confusion
C. Positive cold agglutinin test
D. Splenomegaly
E. Endocarditis
F. Chest radiographic findings of single "circumscribed" lesions

1. *Mycoplasma pneumoniae*
2. *Chlamydia pneumoniae* (TWAR)
3. *Chlamydia psittaci*
4. *Legionella pneumophila*
5. *Francisella tularensis*
6. *Coxiella burnetii*

Question 16.18. Match the patient characteristics to the viral pneumonias with which they are most likely to be associated:

A. Organ transplantation recipients
B. Children
C. Military recruits
D. Debilitated elderly patients

1. Influenza virus
2. Respiratory syncytial virus
3. Adenovirus
4. Cytomegalovirus

Question 16.19. Which of the following condition(s) have been recognized as risk factors for nosocomial pneumonia?

A. Acute illness (shock or hemorrhage)
B. Coexisting illness
C. Therapeutic interventions
D. Impaired nutritional status

Question 16.20. The most common cause of nosocomial pneumonia in ventilated patients is:

A. *Staphylococcus aureus*
B. *Escherichia coli*
C. *Haemophilus influenzae*
D. *Pseudomonas aeruginosa*

Question 16.21. Which of the following sites is NOT a common site for secondary spread and growth of mycobacteria in a patient with *Mycobacterium tuberculosis* pneumonia?

A. Apex of the lung
B. Renal parenchyma
C. Pericardium
D. Growing end of long bones

Question 16.22. The rate of developing pulmonary disease within 2 years following primary infection with *Mycobacterium tuberculosis* in a normal host is:

A. 1%
B. 5%

C. 10%
D. 25%

Question 16.23. **Which of the following statements is/are correct concerning the clinical features of *M. tuberculosis* pneumonia?**

A. Hemoptysis is most often seen as a result of the tuberculous pneumonic process.
B. Culture of pleural fluid has a yield of 75–80% in patients with tuberculous pleural effusion.
C. Pleurisy is a common finding, particularly in the presence of a pleural effusion.
D. Elderly patients will usually have more dramatic symptoms due to their impaired immune system and higher mycobacterial load.

Question 16.24. **A PPD skin test of 10 mm would be indicative of tuberculous infection in patients with which of the following condition(s)?**

A. Intravenous drug user
B. Haitian-born immigrant
C. Nursing home resident
D. Patient who has had ileal bypass surgery
E. Malnourished patient

Question 16.25. **Match the numbered tuberculosis chemotherapeutic agents listed below with their corresponding bactericidal activity:**

A. Rifampin
B. Isoniazid (INH)
C. Streptomycin
D. Pyrazinamide (PZA)

1. Bactericidal against slow-growing intracellular mycobacteria.
2. Bactericidal against actively growing extracellular mycobacteria, slow-growing intracellular mycobacteria, and slow-growing extracellular mycobacteria.
3. Bactericidal against actively growing extracellular mycobacteria.
4. Bactericidal against actively growing extracellular mycobacteria and slow-growing intracellular mycobacteria.

Question 16.26. **In which of the following way(s) does pulmonary disease caused by mycobacteria other than tuberculosis (MOTT) organisms differ from that caused by *M. tuberculosis*?**

A. Lung cavities caused by MOTT are often thin-walled with little surrounding infiltrate.
B. Bronchogenic spread is more common in MOTT.
C. Pleural disease is less common in MOTT.
D. Preexisting chronic pulmonary disease is more common in MOTT.

Question 16.27. **Which of the following clinical findings is sufficient to make a diagnosis of MOTT infection?**

A. Cavitary lung disease in an immunocompetent patient with sputum samples positive for acid-fast bacilli.
B. Immunocompetent patient with chronic pulmonary disease who has a single sputum sample positive for MOTT; subsequent sputum samples are negative.
C. Immunocompetent patient with noncavitary infiltrate with 3 sputum samples positive for MOTT; sputum samples taken after regimen of bronchial hygiene are negative.

D. HIV-infected patient with diarrhea for 1 week and two stool specimens positive for *Mycobacterium avium* complex (MAC).

Question 16.28. **Which of the following statements is/are correct regarding pulmonary disease due to *Histoplasma capsulatum*?**

A. Most primary pulmonary infections with *H. capsulatum* are either asymptomatic or minimally symptomatic.
B. Progressive dissemination of histoplasmosis is usually seen only in patients with decreased cell-mediated immunity.
C. Biopsy specimens from immunocompromised patients with disseminated histoplasmosis show large areas of granulomas with multiple organisms.
D. In immunosuppressed patients, development of disseminated histoplasmosis can result from either new exposure to the fungus or reactivation of previously dormant foci of infection.

Question 16.29. **The most useful serologic test for diagnosing acute infection with *Histoplasma capsulatum* is:**

A. Complement fixation
B. Immunodiffusion
C. Histoplasmin skin test
D. Histoplasma polysaccharide antigen

Question 16.30. **Which of the following statements is/are correct regarding infection with *Coccidioides immitis*?**

A. The most common chest radiographic finding is a progressive upper lobe infiltrate.
B. Like other fungi, serologic testing for diagnosis of coccidioidomycosis is not well developed and of little benefit in acute cases of infection.
C. Coccidioidomycosis is much easier to treat in immunocompromised patients than other dimorphic fungi.
D. Coccidioidal meningitis requires both intravenous and intrathecal amphotericin B for adequate treatment.

Question 16.31. **Which of the following fungal diseases does not usually present as a primary pulmonary disease?**

A. Blastomycosis
B. Cryptococcosis
C. Sporotrichosis
D. Paracoccidioidomycosis
E. Histoplasmosis

ANSWERS

Answer 16.1. **A, B, C, D - True**

It has been estimated that there are one million cases of community-acquired pneumonia requiring hospitalization in the U.S. each year, at an estimated cost of 4 billion dollars. Pneumonia is the sixth leading cause of death in this country, with a mortality rate of 13.4 per 100,000. Nosocomial, or hospital-acquired, pneumonia occurs yearly in at least 275,000 individuals, and is the most important hospital-acquired infection because it is associated with the highest morality rate of any nosocomial infection. Most nosocomial pneumonias are bacterial in origin, although hospital-acquired viral infections can occur.

Reference: page 424

Answer 16.2.   **All are correct**

Certain populations are at increased risk for tuberculosis, particularly African Americans, Hispanics, and immigrants from certain areas. Minority groups now account for more than 71% of all tuberculosis cases in the United States, even though they represent only 26% of the population. As a result of the increasing number of institutionalized elderly individuals, there has been a rise in the occurrence of mycobacterial illnesses in nursing home patients.

Reference: page 424

Answer 16.3.   **A, B, D**

In normal individuals, the paranasal sinuses and the lower respiratory tract (below the vocal cords) are considered sterile, although bacteria can colonize the proximal tracheobronchial tree of smokers and others with impaired host defenses. The nasopharynx is normally colonized with endogenous microflora.

Reference: page 426

Answer 16.4.   **A, C**

The common cold is a symptom complex caused by one of more than 200 viral agents. The most common viral etiologic agent is rhinovirus, of which there are at least 100 types. Smokers have more frequent and more severe viral respiratory illnesses. Therapy with vitamin C is unproven, and has not been shown to improve symptoms or duration of illness.

Reference: page 428

Answer 16.5.   **A**

Bacteriologic studies have shown that sinusitis is caused by *H. influenzae, S. pneumoniae,* and anaerobes, with viruses (rhinovirus, influenza virus, parainfluenza virus) being found occasionally. Less common are *S. aureus,* Gram-negative bacteria, and fungi.

Reference: page 428

Answer 16.6.   **C, D**

Epiglottitis is more common in children than adults, with the incidence greatest between ages 2 and 4. The infection is usually bacterial, with *Haemophilus influenzae* type B being the most common pathogen. Diagnosis is usually made by recognition of the typical signs and symptoms—high fever, drooling, dysphagia, and lethargy; a lateral neck radiograph can confirm the diagnosis when the "thumb sign" of an enlarged epiglottis is seen. Patients should never be examined with a tongue blade, as this may precipitate total airway obstruction. Management is directed initially at maintenance of a patent airway to minimize mortality. With the use of prophylactic artificial airways, mortality in children has fallen below 1%.

Reference: page 429

Answer 16.7.   **D**

Therapy for streptococcal pharyngitis (with penicillin or erythromycin) provides four benefits: reduction in illness duration, avoidance of spread to others, prevention of suppurative complications (such as peritonsillar and retropharyngeal abscess), and prevention of rheumatic fever (but not glomerulonephritis).

Reference: page 430

Answer 16.8. **B**

The three cardinal symptoms of an exacerbation of chronic bronchitis—dyspnea, increased sputum purulence, and increased sputum production—are useful for grading the presence and severity of an infection. Patients with all three symptoms have the most severe exacerbation; approximately 80% of all exacerbations are accompanied by two or three of these cardinal symptoms.

Reference: page 431

Answer 16.9. **B, C, D - True; A, E - False**

Acute respiratory infection from influenza virus results from either type A or B, with the disease from A being generally more severe. Both antigenic drift and waning immunity make influenza a yearly threat, particularly in those with underlying cardiac or respiratory illnesses, the elderly, and pregnant women. Epidemics occur yearly in the late fall and extend into the early spring. Influenza A can coexist with other viral infections including respiratory syncytial virus and parainfluenza virus, particularly in the elderly. If an epidemic of influenza A develops in a closed environment among nonimmunized patients, antiviral therapy should be given along with vaccination, and antiviral therapy is continued for 2 weeks, until the vaccine takes effect.

Reference: page 432

Answer 16.10. **D**

While bacteria reach the lung by all of the routes listed in the question, aspiration is the major route of acquisition for most forms of pneumonia.

Reference: page 433

Answer 16.11. **A, B, D**

Bacteria reaching the lower airways encounter a variety of defense mechanisms. Nonspecific physical barriers include cough, reflex bronchoconstriction, airway angulation, and the mucociliary escalator. When bacteria have prolonged contact with the tracheobronchial mucosa, as is the case when mucociliary clearance is reduced, the extended length of interaction allows the organism to adhere to the mucosa and colonize. In patients with a tracheostomy, colonization of the lower airways by Gram-negative organisms is correlated with an increase in tracheal cell capacity to bind bacteria, thus increasing the risk of colonization. Endotracheal intubation provides a direct means for colonization by organisms which have colonized the oropharynx. Because the lower airways are normally sterile, there is no "normal flora" to prevent growth of pathogens.

Reference: page 434

Answer 16.12. **A-4, B-1, C-2, D-5, E-3**

Certain organisms are known to predominate in pneumonia diagnosed under specific clinical settings, and these associations should be considered when the settings are encountered. Alcoholics may develop pneumonia with *K. pneumoniae*; those with chronic bronchitis can be infected with *H. influenzae*; cystic fibrosis patients develop infections with *P. aeruginosa*; splenectomized patients become infected by encapsulated bacteria, such as *S. pneumoniae*; and leukemics will present with fungal pneumonias, such as *Aspergillus fumigatus*, especially during periods of neutropenia following chemotherapy.

Reference: page 435

Answer 16.13. **D**

Pneumonia can be caused by a wide variety of pathogens, but the responsible agent will vary depending on the status of the patient's underlying host defenses. The most common bacterial pathogen for community-acquired infection is *Streptococcus pneumoniae* for all types of patients.

Reference: page 437

Answer 16.14. **A, C**

There are 84 different serotypes of *Streptococcus pneumoniae*, but 85% of pneumonias are caused by one of 23 serotypes which are now included in the pneumococcus vaccine. Infection is most common in the winter and early spring, which may relate to the finding that viral illnesses are more common then, and up to 70% of patients have a preceding viral illness. In patients with AIDS, pneumococcal pneumonia with bacteremia is more common than in healthy populations of the same age; however, bacteremia is not associated with a mortality rate higher than that of the general population.

Reference: page 438

Answer 16.15. **B, D**

Infection by *Legionella* species is caused by inhalation of an infected aerosol generated by a contaminated water source. Person-to-person spread has not been documented, nor has infection via aspiration from a colonized oropharynx. In hospitalized patients, the most important risk factor for nosocomial *Legionella* pneumonia is the use of corticosteroids. The urinary antigen test can detect only *L. pneumophila* serotype 1 but has high sensitivity and specificity for this organism, which causes more than 80% of clinically evident *Legionella* infections. Treatment of choice for *Legionella* pneumonia is erythromycin in doses of 500–1000 mg every 6 hours intravenously until fever is gone for 2 days.

Reference: page 440

Answer 16.16. **B - True; A, C, D - False**

When aspiration occurs, the right lung is affected more often than the left because of the relatively straighter takeoff of the right mainstem bronchus. When aspiration occurs outside the hospital, infection is usually with anaerobes that have colonized the mouth. Due to the presence of both aerobes and anaerobes associated with aspiration in the nosocomial setting, treatment should include a second- or third-generation cephalosporin or a combination of clindamycin plus an agent active against enteric Gram-negative organisms. The use of corticosteroids and prophylactic antibiotics is of no proven value in preventing pneumonia after a witnessed aspiration.

Reference: page 441

Answer 16.17. **A-5, B-4, C-1, D-3, E-6, F-2**

Tularemia (caused by *Francisella tularensis*) may cause bloody pleural effusions when pneumonia develops. The presence of mental confusion may suggest the diagnosis of Legionella pneumonia. Up to 75% of patients with *Mycoplasma pneumoniae* infection will have a positive cold agglutination test secondary to an IgM autoantibody directed against the I antigen on the red blood cell. Patients with pneumonia due to *Chlamydia psittaci* will commonly have splenomegaly on physical examination. Endocarditis is a commonly reported finding in patients with Q fever (caused by *Coxiella burnetii*). The atypical chest radiographic pattern of a single "circumscribed" lesion is seen in pneumonia due to *Chlamydia pneumoniae* (TWAR).

Reference: page 445

Answer 16.18.   **A-4, B-2, C-3, D-1**

Immunocompromised hosts, such as those having undergone organ transplantation, are often infected with cytomegalovirus. Respiratory syncytial virus most often affects children, while military recruits are at risk for developing pneumonia secondary to adenovirus. Influenza pneumonia develops in adults, particularly the debilitated elderly.

Reference: page 448

Answer 16.19.   **All are correct**

Risk factors for nosocomial pneumonia can be categorized as being of four types: acute illness (such as ARDS, sepsis, or shock) with alterations of lower airway defense mechanisms; coexisting illnesses, such as diabetes, smoking, cardiac or pulmonary disease, or advanced age; therapeutic interventions, such as nasogastric tubes or endotracheal intubation; and poor nutritional status.

Reference: page 449

Answer 16.20.   **D**

Psuedomonas aeruginosa is the most common cause of nosocomial pneumonia in mechanically ventilated patients, accounting for up to 15% of all cases. The organism colonizes the airway in 40% of all mechanically ventilated patients.

Reference: page 450

Answer 16.21.   **C**

After initial infection with *Mycobacterium tuberculosis* in the lungs, some organisms disseminate via the bloodstream to extrapulmonary sites, where they are contained but may later reactivate. The favored sites for secondary seeding and growth are those with high tissue oxygen content such as the apex of the lung, the renal parenchyma, and the growing end of long bones. Pericardial involvement is rare, and is usually due to invasion from a mediastinal lymph node.

Reference: page 458

Answer 16.22.   **B**

About 5% of patients with primary infection from *M. tuberculosis* will not be able to contain the organism and will develop progressive primary disease within 2 years of infection. Rates of 7–8% (or higher in some series) may be seen in patients with HIV infection.

Reference: page 458

Answer 16.23.   **C**

Hemoptysis can be the result of tuberculous pneumonia but is more commonly due to cavitary disease or rupture of an artery in an old tuberculous cavity. Because most of the pleural fluid in cases of *M. tuberculosis* pneumonia is inflammatory rather than infectious, not many organisms are present, and culture of the pleural fluid yields the tubercle bacillus in no more than 20–40% of cases. Pleuritic chest pain is a common finding, especially in the presence of pleural effusions. The elderly generally have less dramatic symptoms than do younger patients.

Reference: page 459

Answer 16.24. **All are correct**

A PPD reaction of 10 mm or more is defined as positive in patients who are foreign born from high-prevalence countries; intravenous drug users; residents of chronic care facilities or correctional institutions; and patients with medical conditions that increase the risk of tuberculosis, such as malnutrition and previous ileal bypass surgery.

Reference: page 461

Answer 16.25. **A-2, B-4, C-3, D-1**

Rifampin is rapidly bactericidal against tubercle bacilli that exist in any of the three populations present in the body: actively growing extracellular organisms, slow-growing intracellular (in macrophages) organisms at acid pH, and slow-growing extracellular organisms. Isoniazid (INH) is bactericidal against the first two of these populations; streptomycin kills only actively growing extracellular bacteria; while pyrazinamide (PZA) kills slow-growing intracellular bacteria.

Reference: page 461

Answer 16.26. **A, C, D**

Pulmonary disease caused by mycobacteria other than tuberculosis (MOTT) appears radiographically similar to tuberculosis, but may differ in that cavities are often thin-walled with little surrounding infiltrate. In addition, bronchogenic spread is unusual, pleural disease is uncommon, and preexisting chronic pulmonary disease is often present.

Reference: pages 462, 463

Answer 16.27. **D**

The diagnosis of MOTT infections is difficult because isolation of the organisms from sputum is not sufficient to establish infection. A diagnosis of pulmonary disease by MOTT is made by having a compatible clinical picture and radiograph in a patient with repeated isolation of organisms from sputum or with evidence of tissue invasion by biopsy. If cavitary disease is present, the diagnosis can be made by finding the organisms on two or more sputum samples, provided that other diagnoses have been excluded. If cavitary disease is absent, the diagnosis requires the above findings plus a failure to convert sputum samples to negative with either bronchial hygiene or two weeks of specific drug therapy. In the AIDS patient, the recovery of MAC organisms from blood or stool, in a patient with a compatible illness, will establish the diagnosis of disseminated infection.

Reference: page 463

Answer 16.28. **A, B, D**

The vast majority of primary infections with *Histoplasma capsulatum* are either asymptomatic or minimally symptomatic. In patients in whom progressive dissemination of histoplasmosis develops, cell-mediated immunity is either decreased or does not develop at all. Histopathologic examination of affected tissue in immunosuppressed patients reveals complete absence of granulomas, and all that is seen are macrophages containing multiple organisms. Two potential pathogenic mechanisms exist for progressive disseminated histoplasmosis (PDH) seen in immunocompromised patients: progression from primary infection after exposure to the fungus, and reactivation of previously dormant foci of infection after immunosuppression.

Reference: pages 464, 465

Answer 16.29. **D**

Skin testing for the diagnosis of histoplasmosis is useful only for epidemiologic purposes. Of the available serologic tests, complement fixation is the most sensitive; however, it takes 2 weeks or more before a four-fold rise can be demonstrated. Immunodiffusion, although highly specific, is relatively insensitive. The best available test is the measurement of the *Histoplasma* polysaccharide antigen, which is also helpful in following the course of treatment and detecting relapses.

Reference: pages 466, 467

Answer 16.30. **D**

The characteristic pulmonary lesion of coccidioidomycosis is a thin-walled cavity; only rarely will pulmonary disease progress to involve the upper lung zones. Unlike other fungal diseases, serodiagnostic tests are not only diagnostic but frequently produce excellent prognostic information. Coccidioidal infections are much more difficult to deal with than other fungi; in immunocompromised patients, treatment is difficult and generally not successful. Coccidioidal meningitis requires both intravenous and intrathecal administration of amphotericin B for adequate therapy. Studies are currently underway using combination therapy, including the imidazoles, for coccidioidal meningitis.

Reference: pages 469, 470

Answer 16.31. **C**

With the exception of sporotrichosis (caused by *Sporothrix schenckii*), the primary mechanism of infection of the listed fungi is via the lungs; *S. schenckii* may also invade the host via the lungs, but the usual manifestation of the illness is lymphocutaneous.

Reference: page 463

chapter 17

Infectious and Noninfectious Pulmonary Complications in Patients Infected with the Human Immunodeficiency Virus

QUESTIONS

Question 17.1. **The most common disseminated fungal disease found in HIV-infected patients worldwide is:**

A. Histoplasmosis
B. Aspergillosis
C. Cryptococcosis
D. Coccidioidomycosis

Question 17.2. **Regarding the occurrence of *Pneumocystis carinii* pneumonia (PCP) in HIV-infected patients, which of the following statements is/are correct?**

A. Most patients have CD4 counts less than 100 at the time of diagnosis of their first episode of PCP.
B. Most patients with PCP will have an elevated serum lactate dehydrogenase (LDH) level.
C. Arterial blood gases in patients with PCP usually reveal respiratory alkalosis and widened PAO_2-PaO_2 gradient.
D. In patients who have had pentamidine prophylaxis prior to their episode of PCP, the lower lobes are the most frequently involved.

Question 17.3. **When considering fiberoptic bronchoscopy with BAL and/or transbronchial biopsies in patients suspected of having *Pneumocystis carinii* pneumonia (PCP), which of the following statements is/are correct?**

A. Biopsies performed greater than 5 days after initiation of treatment for PCP will rarely demonstrate the organism.
B. Transbronchial biopsies should be more strongly considered in patients receiving prophylaxis or who have unusual chest radiograph findings.
C. Transbronchial biopsies are more sensitive than BAL alone in diagnosing PCP.
D. Patients with PCP have an increased risk of pneumothorax following transbronchial biopsies.

Question 17.4. **The following statements are TRUE or FALSE regarding the treatment of *Pneumocystis carinii* pneumonia (PCP)?**

A. Both trimethoprim/sulfamethoxazole (TMP/SMX) and pentamidine are acceptable as antimicrobial agents for PCP, with recommended length of therapy being 14–21 days for either regimen.

B. 50% of patients started on either TMP/SMX or pentamidine will be forced to change to an alternate therapy.
C. If response is not seen in clinical status within 72 hours of initiation of therapy, then alternate medications should be started.
D. Combination therapy using TMP/SMX and pentamidine, when tolerated, is superior to the use of either medication alone.
E. Corticosteroids provide no benefit when added more than 72 hours after beginning anti-PCP therapy.

Question 17.5.   Which of the following statements is/are correct regarding the occurrence of bacterial pneumonia in HIV-infected patients?

A. Ten percent of all pneumonias in HIV-infected patients are due to community acquired bacteria.
B. Clinical presentation of bacterial pneumonia in HIV-infected patients is similar to that in the seronegative population.
C. The most commonly reported bacterial pathogen responsible for pneumonia in HIV-infected persons is *Staphylococcus aureus*.
D. Pneumococcal vaccine is not recommended for use in HIV-infected persons as prophylaxis.

Question 17.6.   Coinfection with HIV and tuberculosis has been seen frequently in all of the following patients groups EXCEPT:

A. Intravenous drug users
B. Foreign-born Cubans
C. Homeless individuals
D. Chronic alcoholics
E. 25- to 44-year-old African Americans

Question 17.7.   Which of the following statements is/are correct regarding the tuberculin skin test in patients with HIV infection?

A. A tuberculin skin test resulting in an induration of 6 mm is considered to be indicative of tuberculosis infection in an HIV-infected person.
B. A negative tuberculin skin test with a positive control rules out tuberculosis infection in an HIV-infected person.
C. The tuberculin skin test is not routinely given to HIV-infected persons unless there is a history of exposure.
D. After close contact with a tuberculous patient, over 25% of HIV-infected patients will develop disease within 5 months.

Question 17.8.   Determine whether the following statements are TRUE or FALSE regarding the clinical features of tuberculosis in HIV-infected patients:

A. *Mycobacterium tuberculosis* is more virulent than other opportunistic infections seen in HIV-infected patients.
B. HIV-infected patients have a low frequency of extrapulmonary involvement.
C. The severity of HIV-induced immunodeficiency may affect the clinical manifestations of tuberculosis.
D. Pleural effusions caused by pulmonary tuberculosis are rare in HIV-infected patients.

Question 17.9.   Anergic HIV-infected patients should be treated with prophylactic therapy under which of the following condition(s)?

A. Close contact with a contagious tuberculous patient.
B. History of 8 mm tuberculin skin test 7 years ago, untreated.
C. Presence of hilar adenopathy on chest radiograph.
D. History of tuberculosis 10 years previously, treated for 3 months only due to patient noncompliance.

Question 17.10. A 24-year-old man presents to the emergency room complaining of fever and cough productive of yellow sputum for 2 weeks. He was diagnosed HIV positive 3 years ago and was hospitalized 8 months ago with *Pneumocystis carinii* pneumonia. He just returned from New York 2 months ago where he was visiting some friends, one of whom had been diagnosed with tuberculosis shortly before he left. The patient's CXR reveals hilar adenopathy and a faint infiltrate in the right upper lobe. His tuberculin skin test shows an induration of 4 mm after 48 hours, and sputum collected for AFB smears are positive. The patient is started on four-drug therapy with INH, rifampin, ethambutol, and PZA. You call the hospital in New York where the contact was treated and are informed that his culture is positive for *M. tuberculosis,* and is resistant to INH. Culture results from your patient also reveal INH resistance. Which of the following should you do regarding your patient's antituberculous therapy?

A. Continue the current therapy as is for a total duration of 24 months.
B. Discontinue the INH and continue therapy with rifampin, PZA, and ethambutol for a total duration of 18 months.
C. Discontinue INH and add streptomycin along with rifampin, PZA, and ethambutol for a total duration of 18 months.
D. Discontinue INH and add streptomycin and amikacin to rifampin, PZA, and ethambutol for total duration of 24 months.

Question 17.11. Which of the following statements is/are correct regarding infection with *Mycobacterium avium* complex (MAC) in HIV-infected patients?

A. MAC usually affects HIV-infected patients with CD4 lymphocyte counts less than 100 cells/mm^3.
B. The respiratory tract is the most common site of dissemination.
C. Diagnosis may be made by demonstration of acid-fast bacilli seen on smear or biopsy.
D. Prophylaxis against MAC is recommended for all HIV-infected patients with fewer than 100 CD4 lymphocytes/mm^3.

Question 17.12. Which of the following condition(s) are diagnostic of clinical cytomegalovirus (CMV) pneumonia in HIV-infected patients?

A. Positive CMV cultures from respiratory secretions or lung tissue.
B. Cytologic or histopathologic demonstration of intranuclear inclusion bodies.
C. Detection of CMV antigen or nucleic acid in tissue.
D. Clinical response to anti-CMV therapy.

Question 17.13. A 32-year-old man, known to be HIV positive for 4 years but without any AIDS-defining illnesses, presents with complaints of fevers, chills, and weight loss for the past 3 weeks, along with cough and mild dyspnea; he denied any mental status changes. Physical examination revealed mild splenomegaly and diffuse lymphadenopathy, primarily in the axillary and femoral areas. Chest radiograph showed a diffuse interstitial infiltrate. CBC reveals a total WBC of 5,900; 73% neutrophils, 11% lymphocytes, and 16% monocytes; the total CD4 lymphocyte count was

245 cells/mm³. The patient currently resides in St. Louis, Missouri, where he has lived for the past 15 years; he has no recent travel history. Which of the following fungi is the most likely etiology of this patient's disease?

A. *Cryptococcus neoformans*
B. *Histoplasma capsulatum*
C. *Coccidioides immitis*
D. *Aspergillus fumigatus*

Question 17.14. Which of the following statements are correct regarding Kaposi's sarcoma (KS) in HIV-infected persons?

A. Kaposi's sarcoma is not considered a true malignancy.
B. The development of KS is dependent on the CD4 lymphocyte count.
C. The diagnosis of pulmonary KS can usually be made with an endobronchial biopsy of a lesion.
D. The presence of pleural effusions is a poor prognostic indicator for KS.

Question 17.15. Which of the following statement is/are correct concerning non-Hodgkin's lymphoma (NHL) in HIV-infected patients?

A. NHL is more likely to occur in HIV-infected patients than in the general population.
B. Like Kaposi's sarcoma, NHL associated with HIV infection occurs mainly in homosexual and bisexual men.
C. HIV-infected patients with NHL are more likely to have dissemination and extra-nodal involvement than immunocompetent patients with NHL.
D. Chemotherapy is associated with increased toxicity in patients with AIDS.

Question 17.16. Determine whether the following statements regarding primary lung cancer in HIV-infected patients are TRUE or FALSE:

A. HIV-infected patients have an increased risk of bronchogenic carcinoma.
B. HIV-infected patients with lung cancer are younger at the time of diagnosis than non-HIV-infected patients.
C. HIV-infected patients with lung cancer have a shorter survival time than non-HIV-infected patients.
D. The predominant cell type of bronchogenic carcinoma in HIV-infected patients is small cell carcinoma.

ANSWERS

Answer 17.1. **C**

The fungus *Cryptococcus neoformans* can be isolated from soil, fruits, and other sources in nature. Due to its worldwide distribution, it is the most common disseminated fungal disease found in HIV-infected patients. Other fungal infections, such as histoplasmosis and coccidioidomycosis, occur in areas where the causative organisms are endemic. Pulmonary aspergillosis is usually diagnosed in the later stages of HIV infection, often in the presence of neutropenia.

Reference: page 488

Answer 17.2. **A, B, C**

Most patients have CD4 counts in the range of 50–75 cells/mm³ at the time of diagnosis of their first episode of PCP and more than 90% of PCP episodes occur when the CD4 count is less than 200 cells/mm³. PCP rarely occurs without an elevation in LDH. Arterial blood gas analysis usually reveals a respiratory alkalosis with a widened alveolar to arterial oxygen pressure difference. Atypical radiographic findings are more commonly found in patients who have other underlying lung disease, have had previous episodes of PCP, or are receiving inhaled pentamidine prophylaxis. Upper lobe disease is more common in patients receiving inhaled pentamidine prophylaxis.

Reference: pages 480–481

Answer 17.3.   B, D are correct

If induced sputum is non-diagnostic for PCP, the next step in diagnosis is bronchoscopy with BAL and/or transbronchial biopsies. Large numbers of *Pneumocystis carinii* cysts and trophozoites remain in lung tissues and pulmonary secretions for weeks to months after the initiation of therapy. Transbronchial biopsies should be more strongly considered in patients receiving prophylaxis or in patients who have unusual chest radiographic findings, as the *Pneumocystis carinii* burden may be less in these patients. Transbronchial biopsies obtained during bronchoscopy have a sensitivity and specificity similar to that of BAL alone; when both BAL and transbronchial biopsies are performed, the sensitivity approaches 100%. Estimates of the incidence of pneumothorax requring a chest tube after transbronchial biopsies in patients suspected of having PCP are up to 5%.

Reference: page 481

Answer 17.4.   A, B, E - True; C, D - False

In patients clinically suspected of having PCP, there are two possible first line antibiotic agents from which to choose, those being trimethoprim-sulfamethoxazole (TMP/SMX) and parenteral pentamidine isethionate. The recommended length of therapy for both medications is 14–21 days. Both medications are associated with significant and potentially life-threatening side effects; in numerous studies, approximately 50% of the patients in whom therapy was initiated with one medication were forced to change to an alternate therapy. It is common for patients who ultimately recover from PCP to deteriorate during the initial 2–3 days of treatment. With this in mind, it has been recommended that alternate therapy should not be started until the patient has received at least 5–7 days of therapy. Combination therapy using TMP/SMX and pentamidine together is not superior to the use of either medication alone. Although the use of corticosteroids clearly reduces the likelihood of death, respiratory failure, or deterioration of oxygenation in patients with moderate to severe PCP, no benefits from the addition of corticosteroids have been found when the corticosteroids were added greater than 72 hours after the start of antipneumocystis therapy.

Reference: pages 481–482

Answer 17.5.   A, B

Up to 10% of all pneumonias in HIV-infected patients are due to community-acquired bacteria. The most common pathogens are the encapsulated organisms *Streptococcus pneumoniae* and *Haemophilus influenzae*. The clinical presentation of acute bacterial pneumonia in HIV-infected patients is similar to that in the seronegative population, with productive cough, fever, and pleuritic chest pain being the most common symptoms. The pneumococcal vaccine is recommended by the Centers for Disease Control for primary prevention of pneumococcal pneumonia in HIV-infected patients, although its efficacy in this population has not been proven.

Reference: page 483

Answer 17.6. **D**

The recent resurgence seen in the rate of tuberculosis cases has been strongly linked to the HIV epidemic. Coinfections with HIV and tuberculosis have been most frequent among foreign-born Haitians and Cubans, 25- to 44-year-old African Americans and Hispanics, the homeless, and intravenous drug users.

Reference: page 483

Answer 17.7. **A, D**

The Centers for Disease Control recommends that all HIV-infected persons receive a tuberculin skin test, regardless of their exposure history. A tuberculin skin test resulting in an induration of 5 mm or more is considered positive and indicative of tuberculous infection in individuals coinfected with HIV. A negative tuberculin skin test, even with positive controls, does not definitively rule out tuberculosis, but does make infection less likely. After close contact with a tuberculous patient, 37% of HIV-infected patients develop disease within 5 months.

Reference: page 484

Answer 17.8. **A, C - True; B, D - False**

Tuberculosis can occur at any stage of HIV infection; *Mycobacterium tuberculosis* is more virulent than other HIV-related opportunistic pathogens (e.g., *Pneumocystis* or cytomegalovirus) and tends to cause disease earlier in the natural history of HIV infection. HIV-infected patients have a high frequency of extrapulmonary involvement, often with concomitant pulmonary tuberculosis. Many reports suggest that the clinical and radiographic manifestations of tuberculosis may vary with the severity of HIV-induced immunosuppression. In patients with less advanced HIV infection, extrapulmonary tuberculosis is uncommon, tuberculin skin tests are usually positive, and chest radiograph findings are often suggestive of reactivation tuberculosis with upper lobe infiltrates and cavitations. In contrast, patients with advanced HIV infection or AIDS tend to have frequent extrapulmonary disease, negative tuberculin skin tests, and chest radiographic findings typical of primary tuberculosis, with hilar adenopathy and interstitial or miliary infiltrates. Pleural effusions are quite common in HIV-infected patients with tuberculosis and have been reported in 11–29% of cases.

Reference: pages 484–485

Answer 17.9. **All are correct**

Prophylaxis with INH is recommended for all HIV-infected patients with a positive tuberculin skin test, regardless of age, unless specifically contraindicated. Anergic HIV-infected patients who have (a) close contacts with contagious tuberculous patients, (b) previously untreated positive tuberculin skin test, (c) chest radiographic findings suggesting previous untreated tuberculosis, or (d) a history of inadequately treated tuberculosis should receive INH prophylaxis as well.

Reference: page 486

Answer 17.10. **B**

HIV-infected patients with either INH or rifampin resistance should be treated with INH or rifampin (whichever has activity against the resistant organism), PZA, and ethambutol for 18 months or 12 months after cultures have converted to negative, whichever is longer.

Reference: pages 485–486

Answer 17.11.   **A, D**

HIV-infected patients with advanced disease and CD4 lymphocyte counts below 100 cells/mm^3 have a unique predisposition for developing MAC infection. Current knowledge suggests that the intestinal tract is a more common site of dissemination than is the respiratory tract. The demonstration of acid-fast bacilli on smear or biopsy is not sufficient for diagnosis of MAC because these organisms may be *M. tuberculosis* or other mycobacteria. All HIV-infected patients with fewer than 100 CD4 lymphocytes/mm^3 should receive prophylaxis against MAC. Rifabutin, 300 mg orally once a day, is the recommended regimen, because it reduces the frequency of disseminated MAC infections in patients with AIDS.

Reference: page 487

Answer 17.12.   **D**

Cytomegalovirus (CMV) is a human herpesvirus that infects 50–95% of the general population by age 40. While CMV infection is usually asymptomatic in immunocompetent patients, it can cause severe end-organ disease in patients with HIV infection. While CMV is frequently isolated from respiratory secretions of HIV-infected patients with pneumonia, its role as a pathogenic organism is controversial. CMV is commonly isolated from the respiratory secretions of patients with concomitant PCP or *S. pneumoniae* pneumonia, and patients recover with treatment of the pathogens without specific anti-CMV therapy. CMV is the sole pathogen in only 4% of all episodes of pneumonia in HIV-infected patients. While a diagnosis of CMV pneumonia may be enhanced by several findings, such as *(a)* positive CMV cultures from respiratory secretions or lung tissue, *(b)* cytologic or histopathologic demonstration of pathognomonic cells with intranuclear inclusion bodies, *(c)* detection of CMV antigen or nucleic acid in tissue, and *(d)* absence of other pathogenic organisms, only a clinical response to anti-CMV therapy confirms the diagnosis.

Reference: pages 487–488

Answer 17.13.   **B**

Symptoms of disseminated histoplasmosis in HIV-infected patients include fevers, chills, and weight loss, often lasting for weeks. Cough and dyspnea are present in 50% of patients; hepatosplenomegaly and lymphadenopathy are present in one-third of cases. Diffuse interstitial infiltrates are the most common chest radiographic abnormalities. This patient lives in an area endemic for histoplasmosis; in areas of high endemicity, disseminated histoplasmosis has been reported to be the second or third most frequent opportunistic infection in HIV-infected patients. Cryptococcus most commonly presents as meningitis, and most often infects HIV-infected patients with CD4 counts below 100/mm^3. Coccidioidomycosis is rarely seen outside its area of endemicity, and this patient has no recent travel history. Aspergillosis is not a frequent opportunistic infection in HIV-infected patients until the advanced stages where neutropenia may be present.

Reference: pages 489–490

Answer 17.14.   **A, D**

Kaposi's sarcoma (KS) is no longer considered a true malignancy, but rather is classified as a proliferative hyperplasia secondary to poor control and regulation of growth factors. The development of KS does not depend directly on the CD4 count. It occurs at a constant rate in patients who are at least 1–2 years post-HIV infection, and the incidence does not increase as the immune system declines. The diagnosis of pulmonary KS is usually made by demonstrating characteristic bright red endobronchial lesions during bronchoscopy. Endobronchial and transbronchial biopsies have a poor diagnostic yield, as a larger segment of tissue than that provided by bronchoscopic forceps is necessary for pathologic diagnosis. The presence of pleural effusions or CD4 counts below 100 predict a poor survival.

Reference: page 492

Answer 17.15.   **A, C, D**

Non-Hodgkin's lymphoma is 60 times more likely to occur in an HIV-infected individual than in the general population. Unlike Kaposi's sarcoma, NHL does not occur in any specific subgroup of HIV-infected patients. Disseminated disease and extranodal involvement are more frequent in the HIV-infected patient than in the immunocompetent patient. Chemotherapy is associated with an increased toxicity in patients with AIDS.

Reference: page 492

Answer 17.16.   **B, C - True; A, D - False**

Epidemiologic studies have not shown an increased risk of bronchogenic cancer in patients infected with HIV. However, HIV-infected patients with lung cancer have been found to be younger and have a shorter survival time than non-HIV-infected patients with primary lung cancer. The predominant cell type of bronchogenic carcinoma in HIV-infected patients is adenocarcinoma.

Reference: page 492

chapter 18

Diseases of the Pleura, Mediastinum, Chest Wall, and Diaphragm

QUESTIONS

Question 18.1.   A 47-year-old male migrant worker comes to the clinic for evaluation of increasing shortness of breath. He smokes two packs of cigarettes per day. Recently he had dyspnea on exertion and now it occurs at rest and he has developed pleuritic chest pain. An arterial blood gas reveals a PaO_2 of 70. A chest x-ray reveals a large right pleural effusion. A thoracentesis demonstrates 550 WBCs with 2 PMNs and 98 lymphs. The LDH pleural fluid/serum ratio is 0.8 and the total protein pleural fluid/serum ratio is 0.9. PPD is nonreactive. Regarding the effusion, which of the following is correct?

A. The majority of tuberculous effusions demonstrate glucose levels below 60 mg/dl, adenosine deaminase (ADA) levels below 70 U/liter, and gamma interferon levels below 2.5 U/ml.
B. Cultures of pleural fluid are positive in the majority of cases of tuberculous pleuritis.
C. A negative PPD in tuberculous pleuritis is thought to be secondary to sequestration of sensitized lymphocytes in the pleural space
D. Pleural fluid AFB stains and cultures are superior to stains and cultures of pleural biopsies in diagnosing pleural tuberculosis

Question 18.2.   A 60-year-old man underwent surgery for repair of a diaphragmatic hernia. Three days later he developed gradually increasing dyspnea, and chest films revealed a new left pleural effusion. A ventilation perfusion scan was normal. A thoracentesis was done, yeilding a white, milky exudate, and the lab reports a triglyceride level of 150 mg/dl in the pleural fluid. Regarding the new pleural effusion, which of the following is correct?

A. Of nontraumatic causes, the most common etiology is fibrosing mediastinitis.
B. Triglyceride levels below 30 mg/dl are characteristic of chylous effusions.
C. Chemical pleurodesis should not be attempted in this man because of lymphatic communications beyond the pleura.
D. The primary danger to patients with this condition is malnutrition.

Question 18.3.   A 48-year-old woman develops acute shortness of breath with chest pain and is brought to the emergency room. A chest film reveals a large right pneumothorax without any midline shift. In the evaluation of a pneumothorax, which of the following is correct?

A. If the pneumothorax is spontaneous, the patient can expect a recurrence in 5 years to exceed 50%.

B. Pleurodesis with bleomycin in primary spontaneous pneumothorax has been shown to be effective.

C. With recurrence of a pneumothorax after chemical pleurodesis, thoracoscopy is indicated, as the likelihood of another recurrence exceeds 80%.

D. Among the bacterial pneumonias, *Streptococcus pneumonia* is most commonly associated with a pneumothorax.

Question 18.4. A 52-year-old man is seen for a routine annual physical exam. A screening chest x-ray reveals a "fullness" of the superior mediastinum. He is a non-smoker and denies any weight loss but has experienced a slight nonproductive cough. Subsequently a CT scan of the chest reveals a 6-cm density above the aortic arch. Regarding the possible etiologies, which of the following is correct?

A. About 20% of mediastinal teratomatous neoplasms are malignant and 90% are located in the anterior mediastinum.

B. Thymic tumors are best treated with radiation and are associated with Guillain-Barré syndrome in 40%.

C. Approximately 90% of testicular germ cell tumors are associated with elevated human chorionic gonadotropin.

D. When the mass extends into the neck, an intrathoracic goiter is diagnosed with the aid of an elevated serum TSH level.

Question 18.5. A 68-year-old male smoker is evaluated for chronic pleuritic chest pain. Chest films reveal a 3-cm pleural density with an associated small effusion. His prior occupation included working in a ship's engine room for 7 years. A thoracentesis revealed a lymphocytic exudate, and subsequently a pleural biopsy was performed, demonstrating only chronic inflammation. At this point in the patient's workup, which of the following is the correct statement?

A. A mesothelioma will stain positive for periodic acid/schiff (PAS) stain as it is a variant of adenocarcinoma.

B. The prognosis with malignant mesotheliomas is favorable because of slow growth and the low potential for metastasis.

C. Pleural biopsies are usually diagnostic in mesotheliomas when combined with cytology from the pleural effusions.

D. Hypertrophic pulmonary osteoarthropathy (HPO) occurs in about 20% of localized benign pleural mesotheliomas.

Question 18.6. An 18-year-old man sustained a crush injury to the chest in an automobile accident. Twenty-four hours after admission a chest film revealed a density consistent with a pulmonary contusion and a pleural effusion. The patient has no past medical history. Which of the following is correct regarding the new pleural effusion?

A. If the thoracentesis fluid is grossly bloody, it can be considered to be from the pleural space if it does not clot.

B. Treatment in this patient is to perform repeated thoracenteses only if symptomatic, to allow the source of bleeding to heal.

C. The physician should allow the body to resorb the blood from a hemothorax as there are few complications as long as there is no infection or hypoxia.

D. A hemothorax can be diagnosed only when the hematocrit of the pleural fluid equals that of the serum.

Question 18.7. A 30-year-old man with a long history of seizures is brought to the emergency room in status epilepticus. Benzodiazepines are given intravenously and the seizures stop. Subsequently the patient becomes apneic and intubation becomes necessary. Attempts at endotracheal tube placement are difficult, and blood is soon noted in the posterior pharynx. Almost immediately the face and neck begin to swell. Crepitations are felt in the neck. In the evaluation of this patient which of the following is correct?

A. The physician should consider anaphylaxis as the most likely etiology of the edema and administer epinephrine.
B. A crunching or clicking noise synchronous with the heartbeat is present in about 50% of cases.
C. A high inspired partial pressure of oxygen may make the problem worse.
D. Surgery is usually required emergently to avoid further complications.

Question 18.8. Regarding the chest wall and the diaphragm, match the following numbered disease or condition with the best lettered definition or statement (answers are used only once).

1. Ankylosing spondylitis
2. Pectus carinatum
3. Kyphoscoliosis
4. Phrenic nerve paralysis
5. Eventration
6. Flail chest

A. Paradoxical diaphragm movement
B. Inspiration aggravates this condition
C. Pseudodiaphragmatic paralysis by chest x-ray
D. Associated with upper lobe fibrosis
E. CPAP is the initial choice of therapy
F. 50% are associated with congenital atrial or ventricular septal defects.

Question 18.9. A 55-year-old man is brought to the emergency room after being found lying in an alley with several empty wine bottles beside him. Upon arrival at the emergency room, the patient is dyspneic and his SaO_2 is noted to be 82%. Chest x-rays reveal a large right lower lobe infiltrate with an associated pleural effusion. His total WBC count is 22,000/mm^3. A thoracentesis reveals turbid fluid with a pleural fluid to serum LDH ratio of 10 and a pleural fluid pH of 6.8. In the management of this patient, which of the following is correct?

A. An increased pleural fluid glucose and an LDH level less than 1000 IU/liter indicate a worse prognosis.
B. Less than 20% of culture positive parapneumonic effusions will contain anaerobic organisms.
C. If indicated, instillation of streptokinase should be performed only one time to avoid an allergic response.
D. If left untreated, an empyema necessitatis may develop.

Question 18.10. Match the following lettered pleural disease caused by parasitic, fungal, and acid-fast organisms to the best numbered statement (answers are used only once).

1. Amebiasis
2. Echinococcosis

3. Paragonimiasis
4. Aspergillosis
5. Histoplasmosis
6. Cryptococcosis
7. Tuberculosis
8. Actinomycosis
9. Nocardia

A. Pleural fluid ADA levels >70 U/liter
B. Treatment usually involves observation
C. Purulent fluid with draining sinus tracts treated with trimethoprim and sul-famethoxazole
D. Bone involvement associated with periosteal proliferation; the treatment of choice is penicillin
E. Rupture of "spring water" cyst into the pleural space
F. Treatment includes irrigating the pleural space with amphotericin B and nystatin
G. Most patients have an associated HIV infection
H. "Chocolate-sauce" pleural fluid
I. A pleural fluid glucose <10 mg/dl, an LDH level above 1000 IU/liter, a pH <7.1, associated with increased blood eosinophils

ANSWERS

Answer 18.1. **C**

Tuberculous pleuritis may occur with or without evidence of pulmonary TB. The pleural fluid usually reveals glucose levels above 60 mg/dl, ADA levels above 70 U/liter and γ interferon above 2.5 U/ml. Plural fluid cultures are positive in less than 20% of proven cases. Pleural biopsy stains and cultures are much more sensitive than pleural fluid stains and cultures, and when combined with cultures of the fluid are positive in more than 90% of cases. The proposed reason for a negative PPD is the migration of sensitized lymphocytes from the blood into the pleural space.

Reference: pages 507–508

Answer 18.2. **D**

Chylothorax is caused by rupture of the thoracic duct into the pleural space. The most common cause is trauma, including surgery involving the mediastinum. Among non-traumatic causes, tumors (including lymphoma) are the most common. Triglyceride levels above 50 mg/dl are typical in chylous effusions. The primary concern with chylous effusions is malnutrition, due to leakage of lymphatic fluid into the pleural cavity and repeated thoracentesis. Multiple thoracentesis may also decrease the number of circulating lymphocytes. Effective treatment includes talc pleurodesis, surgical ligation proximal to the leak, pleuroperitoneal shunts, and irradiation for mediastinal tumors.

Reference: pages 517–518

Answer 18.3. **C**

A pneumothorax is the presence of air in the pleural space caused by trauma or occurring spontaneously. A spontaneous pneumothorax has been shown to recur between 30 and 50% over a 5-year interval. The tetracycline class of antibiotics as well as talc have been shown to be effective with spontaneous pneumothorax, but bleomycin has not.

Staphylococcus aureus is the most commonly associated pathogen when pneumonia and a pneumothorax occur simultaneously. Recurrent pneumothoraces are common after failed initial pleurodesis and a more definitive procedure, thoracotomy or thoracoscopy, is indicated in such cases.

Reference: pages 519–520

Answer 18.4.   **A**

Masses of the mediastinum are divided based on location into the anterior, middle, and posterior compartments. Thymomas are the most common adult mediastinal masses and the preferred treatment is surgical resection. About 25% of thymic tumors are malignant and approximately 40% of thymic tumor patients have myasthenia gravis. Germ cell tumor patients have elevated β-HCG in 30% of cases, while α-fetoprotein levels are elevated in as many as 80%. Goitrous thyroid tissue found substernally, which may first become symptomatic by compressing the trachea, is best diagnosed by demonstrating uptake on an Iodine-131 scan. Mediastinal teratomas are malignant in 20% of cases, and almost always are in the anterior mediastinum.

Reference: pages 520–522

Answer 18.5.   **D**

Mesotheliomas arise from cells that line the pleural cavity; the cells stain negative for PAS. The prognosis of malignant mesotheliomas is poor, with a median survival of about 12 months. Diagnosis is usually only made after an open procedure (thoracoscopy). About 20% of localized benign mesotheliomas have HPO, and about 4% have symptomatic hypoglycemia.

Reference: pages 512–513

Answer 18.6.   **A**

Blood in the pleural space is rapidly defibrinated and does not clot, which differentiates it from a traumatic tap. Most hemothoraces are the result of trauma and are considered to be present when the pleural fluid hematocrit is at least 50% of the serum hematocrit. Patients with traumatic hemothoraces should be managed with a chest tube to allow assessment of persistent hemorrhage and for decisions about potential thoracotomy. Blood is highly fibrogenic and should be removed from the pleural space by a chest tube if the volume of blood is significant. Occasionally the patient may require an open thoracotomy for further evaluation and therapy to avoid "trapped lung." Infections occur more frequently if there is blood in the pleural space.

Reference: page 518

Answer 18.7.   **B**

Pneumomediastinum is the presence of air in the interstices of the mediastinum as the result of alveolar rupture with dissection; perforation of the trachea, esophagus, or main bronchi; or the dissection of air from the abdomen or the neck into the mediastinum (as occurred in this case with trauma from a laryngeal blade). The syndrome may be manifest by a clicking noise with each heartbeat ("mediastinal crunch"). High FiO_2 will help resolve the mediastinal air by creating a diffusion gradient with the blood. Surgery is seldom indicated unless complications such as mediastinitis, vascular compromise, or persistent air leak occur.

Reference: pages 530–531

Answer 18.8.   **1-D; 2-F; 3-E; 4-A; 5-C; 6-B**

Ankylosing spondylitis is an inherited arthritic condition involving the spinal column and is manifest in the lungs in some patients as upper lobe fibrosis. Pectus carinatum is a forward protrusion of the sternum (the opposite of pectus excavatum). Kyphoscoliosis affects the thoracic spine by excessive anteroposterior and lateral curvature, with a resultant restrictive ventilatory impairment leading to alveolar hypoventilation, hypoxia, and eventual pulmonary hypertension. CPAP is recommended as the initial approach to treatment. Phrenic nerve paralysis of any cause will result in ipsilateral hemidiaphragm elevation and a paradoxical movement. Eventration presents as an uneven hemidiaphragm found on chest films noted as "lumpy-bumpy" in appearance. A flail chest is the result of multiple rib fractures that is manifest as paradoxical movement of a part of the chest wall with inspiration and expiration. Vigorous inspiration attempts increase the abnormal chest wall motion.

Reference: pages 531–535

Answer 18.9.   **D**

Parapneumonic effusions are pleural effusions associated with bacterial pneumonias, lung abscess, or bronchiectasis. The parapneumonic effusion is considered complicated if a chest tube for drainage is required. Absolute indications for chest tube insertion are gross pus on thoracentesis, and a positive gram stain of the pleural fluid. Relative indications are a pleural fluid glucose <40 mg/dl, and a pH <7.20 (the latter two in parapneumonic effusions only). More than 1/3 of culture-positive parapneumonic effusions involve anaerobes. Streptokinase (or urokinase) should be offered as the initial choice of therapy in chest tube drainage failures and may be repeated daily for 2 weeks if necessary. Empyema necessitatis is a spontaneous rupture of an empyema through the chest wall due to inadequate drainage.

Reference: pages 505–507

Answer 18.10.   **1-H; 2-E; 3-I; 4-F; 5-B; 6-G; 7-A; 8-D; 9-C**

Many of the fungal and parasitic infections that involve the pleura have common clinical findings, however, some clinical and laboratory clues help to define the correct etiology. Rupture of an amebic abscess into the pleural space may produce a "chocolate-sauce" pleural fluid. A cyst of the liver that ruptures into the thoracic cavity may be due to echinococcosis; the contents of the cyst are usually clear fluid. Paragonimiasis often demonstrates a low pleural fluid glucose, an LDH above 1000 IU/liter, a pH >7.1, and increased blood eosinophils.

Aspergillosis may require treatment with intrapleural amphotericin B in some patients. Treatment of primary histoplasmosis is usually observation only when limited to the thorax. Most patients with pleural cryptococcosis have an associated HIV infection. Adenosine deaminase (ADA) levels are useful in diagnosing tuberculous effusions; a level of >70 U/liter is strongly suggestive of a tuberculous effusion. Actinomycosis often involves the bones of the chest wall, and is associated with periosteal proliferation; treatment is with penicillin. Nocardia is a weakly acid-fast-staining organism that occasionally will cause draining sinus tracts of the chest wall. It is treated with sulfa drugs.

Reference: pages 509–510

Chapter 19

Lung Transplantation

QUESTIONS

Question 19.1. Which of the following condition(s) is/are contraindications to lung transplantation?

A. History of medical noncompliance
B. Poor nutritional status (cachexia, obesity)
C. Significant disease of another organ system
D. Active extrapulmonary infection
E. Current use of tobacco

Question 19.2. Patients with which of the following condition(s) would be candidates for single lung transplantation?

A. Idiopathic pulmonary fibrosis
B. Familial pulmonary fibrosis
C. Sarcoidosis
D. Bronchiectasis
E. Cystic fibrosis

Question 19.3. Determine whether the following statements are TRUE or FALSE with regards to pulmonary reimplantation response (PRR) following lung transplantation:

A. The response is characterized by alveolar consolidation, decreased pulmonary compliance, and abnormal gas exchange.
B. Approximately 50% of patients experience some degree of reimplantation injury.
C. Onset usually occurs 36–48 hours after transplantation.
D. The severity is thought to be related to ischemic time and production of free radicals.
E. Hemodynamic monitoring may helpful in avoiding complications from PRR.

Question 19.4. For which of the following organisms has prophylactic therapy NOT been shown to decrease the occurrence of pneumonia in posttransplant patients?

A. *Pneumocystis carinii*
B. *Herpes simplex* virus
C. *Pseudomonas aeruginosa*
D. *Aspergillus fumigatus*

Question 19.5. A 42-year-old man had a right-sided, single lung transplantation for idiopathic pulmonary fibrosis 45 days ago. He did well postoperatively, but required a transfusion of two units of packed red cells due to blood loss. He was discharged on an immunosuppressive regimen consisting of cyclosporine, azathioprine, and prednisone. He presents with a 10-day history of nonproductive cough, fever, and malaise. Vital signs show blood pressure 120/65; pulse 102; respirations 24; temperature 100.0°F. On chest exam he has fine crackles bilaterally. His chest radiograph reveals mild alveolar infiltrates bilaterally. Serum chemistries and blood counts are normal. Initial sputum smears are negative. The patient remains in stable condition, and the following day a fiberoptic bronchoscopy is performed. Results of the transbronchial biopsies reveal characteristic "owl's eyes" inclusion bodies. Which of the following statements is/are correct regarding the initial treatment of this patient?

A. Foscarnet is the drug of choice in this patient.
B. Polyclonal IgG has been shown to improve survival in these patients.
C. It is important to continue this patient's immunosuppressive agents at their current dosages.
D. Ganciclovir is the drug of choice in this patient.

Question 19.6. In the prevention of obliterative bronchiolitis (OB) following lung transplantation, which of the following statements is/are correct?

A. Single drug immunosuppression is adequate to reduce the incidence of OB.
B. Treatment of clinically asymptomatic rejection has not been shown to decrease development of OB.
C. In patients in whom OB develops, retransplantation is associated with a low level of reoccurrence.
D. The use of surveillance transbronchial biopsy may be beneficial in early detection of OB.

Question 19.7. Which of the following statements is/are correct with regards to acute rejection in lung transplant patients?

A. Acute rejection usually occurs between 10–50 days after lung transplantation.
B. Chest radiograph abnormalities are seen in only 25% of cases diagnosed after the first month post-transplantation.
C. Hypoxemia and deterioration in pulmonary function studies are common findings.
D. Acute rejection cannot be differentiated from infection by clinical findings.

Question 19.8. Match the toxicity with the immunosuppressive agent most likely to cause it. Each answer may be used once, more than once, or not at all.

1. Aseptic meningitis
2. Thrombocytopenia
3. Hyperglycemia
4. Nephrotoxicity
5. Increased risk of malignancy
6. Systemic hypertension

A. Cyclosporine
B. Corticosteroids
C. Azathioprine
D. Antilymphocyte globulin
E. Orthoclone (OKT3)

Question 19.9. Which of the following conditions would exclude a potential donor for single lung transplantation?

A. Age 55 years.
B. PaO_2/FiO_2 ratio of 400 on mechanical ventilation with 5 cm H_2O of positive endexpiratory pressure (PEEP).

C. Positive hepatitis B surface antigen.

D. Unilateral lung injury secondary to trauma.

Question 19.10. Which of the following statements is/are correct concerning general postoperative management after single lung transplantation (SLT)?

A. The addition of PEEP following SLT in patients with obstructive lung disease is useful to help keep the newly transplanted lung inflated.

B. Reperfusion pulmonary edema is a common problem following SLT in patients with pulmonary hypertension.

C. While ganciclovir is routinely given in the posttransplant period if the donor was known to be CMV positive, it is not routinely used if just the recipient is CMV positive prior to transplant.

D. Chest physiotherapy is to be avoided in the postoperative period due to the potential for mechanical complications at the anastomosis.

Question 19.11. Which of the following statements is/are correct regarding airway complications following lung transplantation?

A. Anastomotic complications are seen most frequently in *en bloc* double lung transplantation (DLT)

B. Due to the high rate of potential complications, anastomotic strictures always require surgical repair and reanastomosis.

C. Corticosteroid use following lung transplantation has recently been shown to increase the incidence of airway complications and infections.

D. The development of the omental wrap has decreased the amount of airway complications seen with lung transplantation.

Question 19.12. Which of the following factor(s) can predispose a lung transplant recipient to develop cytomegalovirus (CMV) infection?

A. Receipt of blood products from a CMV-positive donor.

B. CMV seropositivity of the recipient before the transplantation.

C. The use of antilymphocyte agents for immunosuppression.

D. High-intensity immunosuppressive therapy.

Question 19.13. Which of the following statements is/are correct regarding fungal infections in lung transplantation recipients?

A. Fungal infections in lung transplant patients are less common than in other solid organ transplants.

B. The mortality of fungal infections in lung transplant recipients is less than 20%.

C. The most common organisms responsible for fungal infections in posttransplant patients are *Aspergillus* and *Candida* species.

D. Early initiation of amphotericin B has been shown to improve survival in the setting of fungal infections in posttransplant patients.

Question 19.14. The leading cause of morbidity and mortality in recipients of lung or heart-lung transplantation is:

A. Infection

B. Airway complications

C. Graft rejection

D. Obliterative bronchiolitis

ANSWERS

Answer 19.1. **All are correct**

To be considered for lung transplantation, patients must be willing to be compliant with the rigorous medical protocols required for success. Patients should maintain an active lifestyle and an acceptable nutritional status as well. They should have untreatable end-stage pulmonary disease and no other significant medical illness. The presence of infection would exclude a patient due to the necessity of immunosuppressive agents used in the posttransplant stages. Obviously, continued tobacco use despite end-stage pulmonary disease would be a contraindication; most transplant centers require a patient to abstain from cigarette smoking 2 years prior to consideration for lung transplantation.

Reference: page 543

Answer 19.2. **A, B, C**

Restrictive parenchymal lung disease is ideal for single lung transplantation. Single lung transplants have been performed for idiopathic and familial pulmonary fibrosis, sarcoidosis, and many other disorders resulting in end-stage fibrotic lung disease. Patients with suppurative pulmonary diseases, such as bronchiectasis and cystic fibrosis, are not candidates for single lung transplantation; once immunosuppressed, the native lung would infect the transplanted lung or lead to systemic infection.

Reference: page 541

Answer 19.3. **A, D, E - True; B, C - False**

Clinically, the pulmonary reimplantation response (PRR) is characterized by new radiographic alveolar and/or interstitial infiltrates, a decrease in lung compliance, and disrupted gas exchange. It is estimated that up to 80% of patients will experience some degree of reimplantation injury. In general, PRR appears in the immediate postoperative period, whereas rejection and infection are more common after the first 24 hours. Animal studies have suggested that the severity of the PRR is related to the ischemic time and may relate to the production of toxic oxygen-free radicals. Since volume overload can compound the PRR, careful monitoring of hemodynamic parameters via pulmonary artery catheter for at least 2–3 days following lung transplantation is helpful.

Reference: page 547

Answer 19.4. **D**

In transplant centers where trimethoprim-sulfamethoxazole prophylaxis is routinely used during the first year posttransplant and reinitiated when immunosuppression is augmented, the incidence of *Pneumocystis carinii* pneumonitis is less than 1%. *Herpes simplex* viral (HSV) pneumonia or disseminated *Herpes simplex* infection has nearly been eliminated in lung transplant recipients because of the routine use of acyclovir prophylaxis. With the use of broad spectrum antibiotic prophylaxis (usually an anti-Pseudomonal cephalosporin and clindamycin) and routine culturing of the trachea of the donor at the time of harvest, the incidence of bacterial pneumonia has been significantly reduced. Although improved survival is seen in patients with *Aspergillus* pneumonia with the early initiation of high-dose amphotericin, there is no recommended prophylactic therapy for this organism at this time.

Reference: pages 551–554

Answer 19.5.   **D**

The presence of "owl's eye" intranuclear inclusions is diagnostic of cytomegalovirus (CMV) infection. Ganciclovir is currently the mainstay of therapy for invasive CMV disease; foscarnet should be reserved for those patients who develop bone marrow or other toxicities due to ganciclovir therapy. CMV-specific or polyclonal IgG in combination with ganciclovir is associated with improved survival in bone marrow transplant recipients with CMV pneumonitis; however, because of the cost of immunoglobulin and the lack of data in solid organ transplant recipients, IgG is often reserved for life-threatening episodes of CMV infection. With any severe CMV infection, a reduction in the level of immunosuppression is recommended.

Reference: pages 551–552

Answer 19.6.   **B, D**

The use of a three drug immunosuppression regimen has been shown to reduce the incidence of obliterative bronchiolitis (OB). No studies have adequately evaluated the question of whether treatment of asymptomatic rejection will prevent the eventual development of OB. Retransplantation for debilitating OB has been performed, but may be associated with rapid recurrence of OB in the new lung graft. Many transplant centers advocate the use of surveillance transbronchial biopsy as an important mechanism of diagnosing early acute rejection and/or infection and in detecting the development of OB.

Reference: page 551

Answer 19.7.   **All are correct**

Acute rejection is a common immunologic response that usually occurs between 10 and 50 days after lung transplantation, and in many patients, two to three episodes occur within the first month. The chest radiograph is usually abnormal during rejection in the first month posttransplantation, but is abnormal in only 25% of cases after the first month. Hypoxemia and a deterioration in pulmonary function studies frequently occur in the setting of acute rejection; although pulmonary function abruptly improves in the early postoperative period, PFT values may continue to improve for 1–3 months. Clinical criteria alone cannot differentiate acute rejection from infection; transbronchial biopsy has a positive predictive value of 69–83% in lung transplant patients with clinical deterioration. A minimum of five transbronchial specimens containing pulmonary parenchyma should be obtained for histologic evaluation.

Reference: pages 549–550

Answer 19.8.   **1-E; 2-D; 3-B; 4-A; 5-C; 6-A**

Aseptic meningitis has been described in patients on OKT3. Thrombocytopenia is often seen with administration of antilymphocyte globulin; toxicity is most severe with the initial dose. Hyperglycemia is a frequent side effect of corticosteroid use. Nephrotoxicity is the major clinical toxic manifestation of cyclosporine use (25–75% of patients); it is dose related and typically reversible. Systemic hypertension is another serious complication from cyclosporine due to a defect in renal sodium excretion. Patients on azathioprine have been shown to have increased risk of developing certain malignancies, particularly lymphomas, skin tumors, and some solid tumors.

Reference: pages 554–555

Answer 19.9.   **C**

The ideal donor for lung transplant procedures should be less than 65 years of age; donors should be less than 45 years of age to be considered for heart-lung transplant. Donor lungs should exhibit adequate oxygenation , typically defined as a PaO_2 above 300 mm Hg on an FiO_2 of 1.0 and 5 cm H_2O of PEEP. For single lung transplantation, unilateral lung injury secondary to trauma does not automatically exclude the contralateral lung from consideration for donation. Patients are not donor candidates if hepatitis B surface antigen or HIV antibody is present.

Reference: pages 544–545

Answer 19.10.   **B**

In patients with obstructive lung disease, PEEP is usually avoided after SLT due to hyperinflation of the native lung, which can compromise the newly transplanted lung. Ganciclovir is administered for CMV prophylaxis if either the patient or the donor is CMV positive prior to surgery. Both postural drainage and chest physiotherapy can be routinely employed without concern about mechanical complications at the anastomotic site. In patients undergoing SLT for pulmonary hypertension, reperfusion pulmonary edema is often severe because nearly all perfusion is going to the newly transplanted lung.

Reference: page 546

Answer 19.11.   **A, D**

Different lung transplant procedures are associated with varying incidences of airway complications. Heart-lung transplants, single-lung transplants, and bilateral sequential lung transplants have fewer anastomotic complications than *en bloc* double lung transplantations. Airway complications have been reduced with the development of the omental wrap and the telescoping anastomotic technique. Anastomotic strictures may be treated with balloon dilation, wire or silastic stent placement, or surgery. While early studies suggested a higher incidence of complications following corticosteroid administration in lung transplant recipients, more recent clinical studies have shown no correlation between early corticosteroid use and airway complications or infections.

Reference: pages 548–549

Answer 19.12.   **All are correct**

Cytomegalovirus (CMV) is the most common cause of infections in the interval between 30 and 60 days postoperatively. Predisposing factors for CMV infection include receipt of blood products or organs from a CMV-positive donor, CMV seropositivity of the recipient before transplantation, the use of an antilymphocyte agent, and high-intensity immunosuppressive therapy.

Reference: page 552

Answer 19.13.   **C, D**

Fungal infections are more common in lung transplant recipients than in those with other solid organ transplants. The overall mortality of fungal infections in lung transplant recipients is reported between 40 and 70%. Most fungal infections are caused by *Candida* or *Aspergillus* species, and over 80% occur within the first 2 months. Improved survival has been achieved with the early initiation of high-dose amphotericin and the reduction of immunosuppressive therapy in cases of aspergillosis; low-dose amphotericin for the first 14 postoperative days has decreased the occurrence of disseminated *Candida* infections.

Reference: pages 553–554

Answer 19.14.   **A**

Infection is the leading cause of morbidity and mortality in recipients of lung or heart-lung transplantation. The lack of lymphatic drainage and nerve supply, impaired mucosal clearance, and immunosuppression lead to a 30–80% risk of developing a major infection within the first 4 months following transplantation.

Reference: pages 551–552

The Critically Ill Patient

chapter 20

General Principles of Managing the Patient with Respiratory Insufficiency

---

QUESTIONS

Question 20.1. **Which of the following statements regarding dyspnea are True or False?**

A. Dyspnea may be absent in some patients with acute respiratory failure.
B. Dyspnea provides a semiobjective parameter of acute respiratory failure in some patients.
C. There is a reasonably good relationship between dyspnea and arterial hypoxemia but a poor relationship between dyspnea and arterial carbon dioxide retention.

Question 20.2. **With regard to arterial hypoxemia, which of the following statements is/are correct?**

A. Arterial hypoxemia may be caused by alveolar hypoventilation alone.
B. The normal alveolar-arterial PaO_2 difference cannot be calculated if a patient is breathing room air.
C. The distinction between ventilation/perfusion mismatch and right to left intrapulmonary shunting can be made by measuring the response to the administration of 100% oxygen.
D. Supplemental oxygen is often ineffective in treating hypoxemia from ventilation/perfusion mismatch.

Question 20.3. **With regard to arterial hypercapnia, which of the following statenents is/are correct?**

A. The quantity of alveolar ventilation necessary to eliminate CO_2 and maintain a normal $PaCO_2$ varies depending on carbon dioxide production.
B. Alveolar hypoventilation can occur because of increased production of carbon dioxide.
C. Alveolar hypoventilation can occur because of a decrease in minute ventilation.
D. Alveolar hypoventilation can occur because of an increase in wasted ventilation.

Question 20.4. **With regard to metabolic and respiratory acidosis, which of the following statements are true or false?**

A. The relationship between $PaCO_2$ and plasma bicarbonate concentrations determine the arterial pH.
B. The relationship between $PaCO_2$ and arterial pH varies depending on the time during which the $PaCO_2$ has increased.
C. For every 10 mm Hg change in $PaCO_2$, the pH changes by approximately .008 in the opposite direction.

D. An acute rise in the $PaCO_2$ from 40 to 60 mm Hg would be expected to cause a decrease in arterial pH to 7.10.

Question 20.5. **With regard to respiratory and metabolic alkalosis, which of the following statements is/are correct?**

A. Alkalosis may predispose to arrhythmias.
B. Alkalosis may cause an increase in cardiac output.
C. Alkalosis may reduce the threshold for seizures.
D. Hypocapnia with or without alkalosis increases cerebral blood flow which may depress the level of consciousness.

Question 20.6. **Which of the following statements regarding measurement of vital capacity and inspiratory force is/are true or false?**

A. The vital capacity is the maximum volume of air that can be exhaled after maximal inspiration.
B. The vital capacity is influenced by the chest wall, the elastic properties of the lung, the caliber of the airways and by the respiratory neuromuscular system.
C. The minimal acceptable vital capacity in most patients is from 10 to 15 ml/kg body weight.
D. A minimal acceptable inspiratory force is -20 cm H_2O in ventilated patients.

Question 20.7. **With regard to the interrelationship of $PaCO_2$ carbon dioxide production and alveolar ventilation, which of the following statements are true or false?**

A. Total minute ventilation is the product of tidal volume and the frequency of the respiratory rate.
B. $PaCO_2$ is related directly to both carbon dioxide production and to alveolar ventilation.
C. Alveolar ventilation is the difference between tidal volume and the wasted or dead space ventilation multiplied by the respiratory rate. Normal values for the fraction of wasted ventilation are .30–.35.

Question 20.8. **With respect to calculations of oxygenation, which of the following statements is/are true?**

A. The partial pressure of oxygen in the alveolus can be calculated from the alveolar gas equation.
B. The alveolar gas equation provides a quantitative assessment of the degree of hypercapnia.
C. If the patient has arterial hypoxemia, but a normal alveolar to arterial oxygen difference, then this finding suggests that the hypoxemia may be secondary to alveolar hypoventilation.
D. If the alveolar to arterial oxygen difference is increased above normal, then this finding indicates that there is an intrapulmonary or intracardiac right to left shunt or mismatching of ventilation and perfusion as an explanation for the defect in oxygenation.

Question 20.9. **With regard to the selection of the type of oxygen delivery device, the choice depends on which of the following factors:**

A. The quantity of oxygen needed
B. The need for precise control of the fraction of inspired oxygen
C. The need for humidification
D. The patient's comfort

Question 20.10.   **With regard to the following statements regarding the advantage of an oral route for endotracheal intubation which statements is/are correct?**

A. A larger-diameter tube can be used.
B. Direct laryngoscopy is not required.
C. It is easier to insert under emergency conditions.
D. The danger of esophageal intubation is avoided.

Question 20.11.   **Which of the following statements about nasal endotracheal tubes is/are correct?**

A. Nasal endotracheal tubes are easier to suction through than oral tubes.
B. Nasal endotracheal tubes are generally more comfortable for the patient.
C. Fiberoptic bronchoscopy can be done more easily through a nasal endotracheal tube than an oral tube.
D. Suctioning may be difficult because of compression or kinking of the endotracheal tube within the nose or the nasal pharynx.

Question 20.12.   **With respect to the general clinical situation in which mechanical ventilation is most commonly used, which of the following statements is/are correct?**

A. Severe hypoxemia, usually due to intrapulmonary shunting of blood
B. Alveolar hypoventilation with progressive respiratory acidosis
C. For respiratory support following major cardiac surgery
D. For patients who require general anesthesia or heavy sedation for diagnostic therapeutic interventions

Question 20.13.   **Which of the following statements regarding important features of volume ventilators are true or false?**

A. The ventilator needs to be able to deliver a wide range of tidal volumes (100–1500 ml)
B. Controls are not needed for adjusting the inspiration/expiration ratio or the inspiratory flow rate
C. The ventilator must have alarms that monitor exhaled tidal volume, inspiratory pressure, and the fraction of inspired oxygen

Question 20.14.   **Match the following characteristic of ventilators with the appropriate type of ventilator support.**

1. Intermittent mandatory ventilation (IMV)
2. Intermittent positive pressure ventilation (IPPV)
3. Positive end-expiratory pressure (PEEP)
4. Continuous positive airway pressure (CPAP)

A. Pleural pressure is negative during inspiration.
B. Moderate to high levels (10–20 cm of H_2O) may be associated with barotrauma and/or a decrease in cardiac output.
C. Pressure support ventilation can be used as an adjunct to assist spontaneous ventilations between the preset ventilator delivered breaths.
D. Spontaneous ventilation is not possible with this mode of ventilation.

Question 20.15.   **Which of the questions about positive end-expiratory pressure are true or false?**

A. PEEP increases intrathoracic pressure and, therefore, reduces return of blood from the venous circulation to the right ventricle.

B. Arterial oxygen tension may improve, even though cardiac output may decline.
C. PEEP may increase intrapulmonary shunt by decreasing blood flow to more normal alveoli and increasing flow to fluid filled or collapsed alveoli.
D. PEEP is equally useful in patients with obstructive as well as restrictive lung disease.

Question 20.16. **With regard to sounding of the high pressure limit alarm during mechanical ventilation, which of the following statements is/are correct?**

A. The high pressure alarm may be exceeded because of disconnection of the ventilator circuit from the endotracheal tube.
B. The high pressure alarm may be exceeded because of obstruction of the endotracheal tube with mucous or blood clot.
C. High pressure alarm may be sounded because of arterial hypoxemia.
D. High pressure alarm may be sounded because of the development of a pneumothorax.

Question 20.17. **When inadequate ventilation is noted (the delivered tidal volume is not being delivered or the patient's chest is not moving), which of the following statements are true or false?**

A. There may be a leak in the ventilator tubing.
B. There may be a leak around the cuff of the artificial airway.
C. The endotracheal tube may have moved approximately above the glottis.
D. There may be a malfunction of the ventilator.

Question 20.18. **When attempting to wean a patient from mechanical ventilation, which of the following statements is/are correct?**

A. The underlying medical or surgical problem that necessitated mechanical ventilation must be resolving.
B. The patient should be awake and reasonably alert.
C. In general, the patient should have a vital capacity greater than 10 ml/kg or a maximum inspiratory pressure of less than -20 cm H_2O.
D. The patient should not require an FIO_2 above 0.3.

Question 20.19. **Which of the following statements about failure to wean from mechanical ventilation is/are correct?**

A. A diminished level of consciousness is an important cause of unsuccessful weaning.
B. The need for nebulized bronchodilators precludes successful weaning from mechanical ventilation.
C. Pulmonary insufficiency is the most common cause for failure to wean from mechanical ventilation.
D. A decrease in mental status in mechanically ventilated patients is usually related to injudicious use of sedatives.

Question 20.20. **With respect to respiratory monitoring, which of the following statements are true or false?**

A. Respiratory monitoring in patients with respiratory failure in the intensive care unit should always include the measurement of respiratory rate and arterial oxygen saturation.
B. Measurement of tidal volume and minute ventilation is useful in most patients being treated for respiratory failure with mechanical ventilation.

C. Respiratory muscle fatigue is often clinically evident because of the development of tachypnea and abdominal paradox.
D. A rise in arterial PCO_2 is an early sign of respiratory muscle fatigue.

ANSWERS

Answer 20.1.   **A-True; B, C-False**

Dyspnea is a subjective finding. There is no clear-cut relationship between dyspnea and specific blood gas abnormalities.

Reference: pages 563–564

Answer 20.2.   **A, C are correct**

The alveolar oxygen difference can be easily calculated if the patient is breathing room air because the fraction of inspired oxygen is known to be .21. Supplemental oxygen is often very effective in treating arterial hypoxemia from ventilation perfusion mismatch whereas it may be relatively ineffective in treating arterial hypoxemia from right to left pulmonary shunting.

Reference: page 565

Answer 20.3.   **A, B, C, D are correct**

There are multiple physiologic mechanisms by which $PaCO_2$ may increase. It is important to be familiar with all of these physiologic mechanisms.

Reference: pages 565–566

Answer 20.4.   **A, B, C-True; D-False**

It is very useful to understand the relationship between $PaCO_2$ and plasma bicarbonate concentrations and to be able to determine whether they reflect acute or chronic changes. An acute rise in the $PaCO_2$ from 40–60 mm Hg would be expected to cause a decrease in arterial pH to approximately 7.24, assuming that the patient's initial pH was normal (pH 7.40).

Reference: page 566

Answer 20.5.   **A, C are correct**

Metabolic alkalosis may cause a decrease in cardiac output and hypocapnia decreases cerebral blood flow; it does not increase cerebral blood flow.

Reference: page 566

Answer 20.6.   **A, B, C, D-True**

All of these answers are correct are very useful to bear in mind when measuring vital capacity in patients in the intensive care unit.

Reference: page 566

Answer 20.7.   **A, C-True; B-False**

$PaCO_2$ is related directly to carbon dioxide production but inversely to alveolar ventilation.

Reference: page 567

Answer 20.8.   **A, C, D-True; B-False**

Answer B is incorrect because the alveolar gas equation provides a quantitative assessment of the degree of hypoxemia. See the text on pages 567 and 568 for further discussion.

Reference: pages 567–568

Answer 20.9.   **A, B, C, D are correct**

These are all important issues in selecting the oxygen delivery device or method for patients with hypoxemia.

Reference: page 568

Answer 20.10.   **A, C are correct**

Direct laryngoscopy is almost invariably required for oral endotracheal intubation. Esophageal intubation may certainly occur under these circumstances as well. See the text on page 568 and the references to recent studies in critically ill patients on the issue of esophageal intubation.

Reference: page 568

Answer 20.11.   **B, D are correct**

Nasoendotracheal tubes are usually more difficult to suction through than oral tubes because they are often smaller in size and because of the compression or kinking of the tube as it passes through the nose and the nasopharynx.

Reference: page 569

Answer 20.12.   **A, B, C, D are correct**

Please see the text on page 570 for further discussion.

Reference: page 570

Answer 20.13.   **A, C-True; B-False**

It is important to adjust the inspiratory and expiratory ratio or the inspiratory flow rate. For example, prolonged expiratory flow rates are needed in patients with airway obstruction such as asthma or chronic obstructive lung disease.

Reference: page 570

Answer 20.14.   **1-C; 2-D; 3-B; 4-A**

Pressure support ventilation is typically used in conjunction with intermittent mandatory ventilation or occasionally on its own in a weaning phase. In the intermittent positive pressure ventilation mode, there is no possibility of spontaneous ventilation. The patient can increase the respiratory rate but will receive the preset tidal volume. Positive end expiratory pressure may be associated with an increased risk for barotrauma particularly when the levels of PEEP are about 10–20 cm H_2O. During spontaneous ventilation with continuous positive airway pressure, pleural pressure is negative.

Reference: pages 570–571

Answer 20.15. **A, B, C-True; D-False**

Answer D is False because PEEP has not been demonstrated to be useful in most patients with acute or chronic obstructive lung disease. The functional residual capacity has already increased in patients with obstructive lung disease.

Reference: pages 571–572

Answer 20.16. **B, D are correct**

The low pressure alarm will be exceeded because of disconnection from the ventilator circuit. The high pressure alarm will not sound if the patient is hypoxemic. The oxygen saturation monitor should alarm if the oxygen saturation falls below a preset level (such as 80% oxygen saturation).

Reference: page 572

Answer 20.17. **A, B, C, D-True**

All the statements are correct. It is very important to know how to recognize inadequate ventilation in a patient who is mechanically ventilated.

Reference: page 573

Answer 20.18. **A, B, C are correct**

Statement D is not correct because it is not necessary that a patient be adequately oxygenated with an FIO_2 as low as 0.3. In general, adequate oxygen with an FIO_2 of 0.5 or less is a reasonable criterion for proceeding to weaning from mechanical ventilation.

Reference: page 573

Answer 20.19. **A, C are correct**

Nebulized bronchodilators can be given to extubated patients. Also, it is possible to give bronchodilators by metered dose inhaler. Decrease in mental status in mechanically ventilated patients is more often than not related to underlying medical problems such as liver disease or uncontrolled infection, less often to the injudicious use of sedatives. See Reference 30 in Chapter 20.

Reference: pages 573–574

Answer 20.20. **A, B, C-True; D-False**

A rise in arterial PCO_2 is actually a relatively late sign of respiratory muscle fatigue. See the text on page 574 as well as Figure 20.7.

Reference: page 574

chapter 21

Acute Hypercapnic Respiratory Failure: Neuromuscular and Obstructive Diseases

QUESTIONS

Question 21.1. Which of the following statements regarding the etiology of neuro-muscular disorders causing acute respiratory failure is/are correct?

A. Guillain-Barré syndrome is a cause of acute respiratory failure.
B. Electrolyte disorders such as hypokalemia and hypophosphatemia may also cause sufficiently severe muscle weakness to cause acute respiratory failure.
C. Neuromuscular blocking agents may be associated with persistent respiratory failure.
D. Organic phosphate poisoning is a neuromuscular cause of acute respiratory failure.

Question 21.2. Which of the following statements regarding Guillain-Barré syndrome are true or false?

A. Approximately 20–30% of patients with Guillain-Barré syndrome require mechanical ventilation.
B. The average duration of mechanical ventilation in Guillain-Barré syndrome dependent on respiratory failure is 4–6 weeks although the range is variable.
C. Characteristically, patients with Guillain-Barré syndrome who require mechanical ventilation have a forced vital capacity in the range of 10–11 ml/kg body weight.
D. Lobar atelectasis and pneumonia may complicate Guillain-Barré syndrome particularly in the early phase of respiratory failure prior to the institution of mechanical ventilation.

Question 21.3. Which of the following statements regarding treatment for respira-tory failure requiring mechanical ventilation in patients with Guillain-Barré syndrome is/are correct?

A. Many experts recommend the use of prophylactic subcutaneous heparin to prevent thromboembolic complications.
B. Psychosocial issues are of relatively minor significance in these patients.
C. Plasmapheresis is of proven treatment value in patients with respiratory failure from Guillain-Barré syndrome.
D. Corticosteroids are of some clinical benefit for treatment of patients with acute res-piratory failure from Guillain Barré syndrome.

Question 21.4. Which of the following questions regarding drug overdoses and acute respiratory failure are true or false?

A. Initial treatment of drug overdose patients in the emergency room usually includes an attempt to remove any unabsorbed drug with emesis or gastric lavage.

B. Activated charcoal no longer is recommended in patients with drug overdose.
C. A decrease in mental status with an associated decrease in normal airway reflexes constitutes an important indication for intubation of patients with drug overdoses.
D. Several drugs have been specifically associated with the development of acute lung injury and noncardiogenic pulmonary edema; these drugs include aspirin, heroin, and ethchlorvynol.

Question 21.5. Which of the following statements regarding acute and chronic respiratory failure from abnormalities of the chest wall is/are correct?

A. Pulmonary hypertension may develop.
B. There may be a relationship between the elevation of pulmonary arterial pressure and the angle of spinal deformity in patients with scoliosis.
C. Ventilation/perfusion mismatching is an important cause of blood gas abnormalities.
D. Positive pressure ventilation is not useful for reversing acute respiratory failure in patients with chest wall abnormalities as a cause of their respiratory failure.

Question 21.6. The following statements regarding chronic obstructive lung disease is/are correct?

A. Primary mechanism of hypoxemia is related to right to left intrapulmonary shunt.
B. Respiratory muscle fatigue may make an important contribution to acute respiratory failure in patients with COPD.
C. A decrease in central ventilatory drive in these patients is completely explained by an acquired, as opposed to a genetic, decrease in ventilatory drive.
D. Central nervous system abnormalities such as decrease in consciousness or even seizures may occur as a major manifestation of acute respiratory failure in COPD.

Question 21.7. Which of the following statements regarding the physical examination for patients with acute respiratory failure and COPD are true or false?

A. Central nervous system examination is important.
B. The degree of pulses paradoxus does not correlate usually with the severity of airway obstruction.
C. Breath sounds are commonly diminished.
D. Supraclavicular and intercostal space muscle retractions do not correlate with increased work of breathing.

Question 21.8. Which of the following statements regarding laboratory evaluation of acute respiratory failure and COPD is/are correct?

A. The electrocardiogram may showing right atrial or right ventricular enlargement is a sign of right heart strain.
B. Polycythemia may be present.
C. Plasma bicarbonate may be elevated.
D. Measurement of arterial pH helps to determine whether the patient's hypercapnia is chronic or acute.

Question 21.9. If a patient with COPD has acute respiratory failure with the following arterial blood gas, pH = 7.28, PCO_2 = 65, PO_2 = 51 on room air, which of the following statements is/are correct?

A. The most important treatment to deliver in patients with decompensated obstructive lung disease is supplemental oxygen therapy.
B. Arterial oxygen tension should be maintained at approximately 60–65 mm Hg.

C. A Venturi device may be more accurate in delivering a precise fraction of inspired oxygen than nasal prongs.
D. It is reasonable to allow the arterial PaO_2 to decline to 45–50 mm Hg in the arterial blood in order to try to prevent the patient from developing progressive hypercapnia and respiratory acidosis.

Question 21.10. Which of the following statements regarding mechanical ventilation for acute respiratory failure and COPD are true or false?

A. Tidal volumes should be set at approximately 7–10 ml/kg body weight.
B. The respiratory rate should be in general set at 15–25/minute.
C. A short inspiratory time is usually desirable to improve the distribution of inspired gas.
D. PEEP of 8–12 cm H_2O should be administered early in the course of the patients ventilatory treatment.

Question 21.11. A 60-year-old gentleman with COPD has been treated with positive pressure ventilation for 4 days. He appears to be ready for weaning from the ventilator. Which of the following questions regarding weaning patients with chronic airway obstruction from mechanical ventilation are true or false?

A. The patient should have a normal $PaCO_2$ before initiation of weaning.
B. There is no evidence that one weaning modality is clearly superior to another weaning modality.
C. Muscle fatigue may occur with prolonged T-piece or CPAP weaning trial
D. Twenty-four month survival rates for patients who develop acute respiratory failure in the presence of COPD range from 35–70%.

Question 21.12. Which of the following statements regarding treatment of acute respiratory failure and COPD is/are correct?

A. Inhaled β_2-adrenergic agonists should be used as a mainstay of treatment.
B. β_2-agonists should always be administered as a metered dose inhaler.
C. Inhaled ipratropium may provide additional bronchodilatation and reduce the volume of secretions.
D. Parenteral glucocorticoids have no proven benefit in acute respiratory failure from COPD.

Question 21.13. Which of the following statements regarding status asthmaticus are true or false?

A. Asthma mortality is on the decline in the United States and worldwide.
B. Physiologically, patients with acute status asthmaticus have both hypoxemia from ventilation/perfusion mismatch as well as an increase in wasted ventilation.
C. Carbon dioxide retention and acute respiratory acidosis indicate that the patient has severe potentially life-threatening asthma.
D. Both metabolic and respiratory acidosis may occur in status asthmaticus.

Question 21.14. A 24-year-old woman with a history of recurrent severe asthma attacks presents to the emergency room with a pulse = 128/min, blood pressure of 160/100 mm Hg, and a respiratory rate of 40/min. Which of the following statements regarding the history and physical examination in status asthmaticus are true or false?

A. Patients with a history of prior severe asthma attacks have a greater likelihood of developing acute respiratory failure.

B. The degree of pulses paradoxus does not correlate with the degree of airway obstruction.
C. Unilateral absence of wheezing may be the result of a pneumothorax or a mucous plug in the large airway.
D. Abnormalities of vital signs are very important in assessing the severity of acute respiratory failure in status asthmaticus.

Question 21.15. **Which of the following questions regarding laboratory evaluation of status asthmaticus is/are correct?**

A. The peak expiratory flow is the most easily obtained pulmonary function test because it does not require a forced exhalation.
B. An FEV_1 of less than 1.5 liters or 40% of predicted value is associated with a poor bronchodilator response, the need for hospitalization, and the likelihood of relapse.
C. Values of arterial PO_2 of less than 50 mm Hg in acute asthma are unusual and suggest that other factors, such as pneumothorax or pneumonia, may contribute to the hypoxemia.
D. A chest radiograph does not need to be obtained routinely in all patients with severe asthma.

Question 21.16. **Which of the following statements regarding airway management in patients with status asthmaticus are true or false?**

A. Nasotracheal intubation may provoke increased bronchial constriction.
B. Sedation and analgesia are usually required immediately after intubation for status asthmaticus.
C. Initial ventilatory management should include setting the tidal volume at 15 ml/kg body weight.
D. Because auto-PEEP is invariably present in status asthmaticus, application of PEEP shortly after intubation should be routinely done in the range of 5–10 cm of H_2O.

Question 21.17. **A 35-year-old gentleman has been admitted to the intensive care unit for treatment of status asthmaticus. Which of the following statements regarding treatment of status asthmaticus is/are correct?**

A. β-adrenergic agonists have the most favorable benefit to risk ratio when they are given by inhalation in status asthmaticus.
B. Treatment with corticosteroids in status asthmaticus is a mainstay of therapy.
C. Aerosols of corticosteroids should be initiated after resolution of the acute phase of status asthmaticus.
D. Antimicrobial agents are of uncertain value in the routine management of acute asthma.

ANSWERS

Answer 21.1. **All are correct**

There is a detailed discussion of neuromuscular respiratory failure in the text.

Reference: page 578

Answer 21.2. **A, B, D-True; C-False**

Most patients with Guillain-Barré syndrome who require mechanical ventilation have a force vital capacity of 5 ml/kg/body weight or less. Note that lobar atelectasis and pneumonia are commonly found in patient with Guillain-Barré syndrome before intubation because the patients often have subclinical aspiration of pharyngeal contents and have not been able to cough and breathe effectively, thus resulting in atelectasis and pneumonia.

Reference: page 573

Answer 21.3. **A, C**

Several studies have shown that psychosocial issues are very important in the management of patients with Guillain-Barré syndrome, particularly since the syndrome occurs acutely in previously health individuals. Secondly, corticosteroids have not been shown to be effective in the treatment of acute respiratory failure with Guillain-Barré syndrome, whereas plasmapheresis is shown to be of value in a prospective, randomized trial.

Reference: page 579

Answer 21.4. **A, C, D-True; B-False**

Activated charcoal is still used to help bind any drug that has not been absorbed in the gastrointestinal tract.

Reference: page 580

Answer 21.5. **A, B, C**

Positive pressure ventilation may well reverse acute respiratory failure in patients with chronic respiratory failure from abnormalities of the chest wall. For example, patients may develop intercurrent bronchitis or pneumonia which will improve with antibiotics, suctioning, and rest with positive pressure ventilation.

Reference: page 581

Answer 21.6. **B, D**

The primary mechanism of hypoxemia in most patients with exacerbated chronic obstructive lung disease is ventilation/perfusion mismatch. This is the reason why low flow oxygen can be usually effective in reversing hypoxemia in exacerbated COPD. Also, a decrease in central ventilatory drive has been shown to be related to genetic factors as well as acquired abnormalities during the course of chronic obstructive lung disease.

Reference: page 502

Answer 21.7. **A, C-True; B, D-False**

The degree of pulsus paradoxus does correlate usually with a severity of airway obstruction, and supraclavicular and intercostal space muscle retractions is a reasonably good clinical sign of increased work of breathing.

Reference: page 583

Answer 21.8. **All are correct**

Reference: pages 583, 584

Answer 21.9. **A, B, C**

The arterial oxygen tension should not decline below 60 mm Hg because the patients pulmonary hypertension and right ventricular workload may increase with a subsequent decline in cardiac output and an increased risk of arrhythmias. If the patient develops progressive hypercapnia and respiratory acidosis with the arterial PO_2 in the range of 60 mm Hg (90% oxygen saturation), then intubation and positive pressure ventilation are indicated.

Reference: page 584

Answer 21.10. **A-True; B, C, D-False**

In terms of the respiratory rate, it should be adjusted according to what is needed to normalize the arterial pH. A short inspiratory time is useful primarily to allow a longer time for expiration, not to improve the distribution of inspired gas. Finally, PEEP should not be administered in most patients with acute respiratory failure from COPD because they already have a high lung volume with an increased functional residual capacity as well as some evidence in most patients of auto-PEEP.

Reference: page 585

Answer 21.11 **B, C, D-True; A-False**

The patient should have a nearly normal pH before initiation of weaning. It is not necessary that the $PaCO_2$ be normal, particularly because the patient may chronically have an elevated PCO_2.

Reference: pages 585, 586

Answer 21.12. **A, C**

β_2-agonists may be more effective in some patients if given by nebulization. One prospective randomized study showed therapeutic benefit of systemic glucorticoids for acute exacerbation of COPD.

Reference: pages 586

Answer 21.13. **B, C, D-True; A-False**

In fact, asthma mortality is on the increase in the United States as well as internationally. The explanation for this increase in mortality is not clear.

Reference: pages 536, 537

Answer 21.14. **A, C, D-True; B-False**

As in exacerbation to COPD, the degree of pulses paradoxus usually does correlate with the severity of airway obstruction.

Reference: page 587

Answer 21.15. **A, C**

An FEV_1 that is less than 750 ml is often associated with a need for hospitalization in acute asthma. Secondly, a chest radiograph should always be obtained in patients with severe asthma to rule out pneumothorax or pneumonia.

Reference: page 588

Answer 21.16. **A, B-True; C, D-False**

Patients with status asthmaticus have a markedly increased functional residual capacity and air trapping. Therefore, their initial tidal volume should not be set at 15 ml/kg/body weight. A lower tidal volume in the range of 6–10 ml/kg is usually more appropriate. Secondly, PEEP should not be used in most patients with status asthmaticus because they already have a high lung volume and because they do have auto-PEEP.

Reference: pages 588, 589

Answer 21.17.   **All are correct**

For a more detailed discussion of therapeutic issues in asthma, please see the discussion on pages 589–591.

Reference: pages 589, 590

chapter 22

Acute Hypoxemic Respiratory Failure: Pulmonary Edema and ARDS

QUESTIONS

Question 22.1. **Which of the following statements regarding the pathogenesis of pulmonary edema is/are correct?**

A. A rise in microvascular hydrostatic pressure in the pulmonary circulation is one important cause of pulmonary edema.
B. A rise in microvascular protein osmotic pressure is another mechanism that may lead to the development of pulmonary edema.
C. An increase in microvascular permeability in the lung is another important physiologic mechanism that may lead to pulmonary edema.
D. Lung lymphatics are important in maintaining normal lung fluid balance only under pathological conditions.

Question 22.2. **Which of the following statements regarding high pressure pulmonary edema is/are true or false?**

A. A modest increase in left atrial pressure (14–20 mm Hg) normally results in the development of mild to moderate interstitial pulmonary edema.
B. As left atrial pressure rises to above 25–30 mm Hg, interstitial fluid normal floods into the distal airspaces of the lung, a pathologic condition that is associated with the development of arterial hypoxemia.
C. The protein concentration of edema fluid in hydrostatic edema is similar to the protein concentration in the plasma.
D. Pleural effusions form in association with hydrostatic pulmonary edema primarily because of the elevation of left atrial pressure in association with the increase in lung water.

Question 22.3. **A 58-year-old gentleman is admitted to the intensive care unit with a presumed diagnosis of acute myocardial infarction with clinical evidence of systemic hypertension and pulmonary edema on chest radiograph. Which of the following statements is/are correct regarding treatment of high pressure cardiogenic pulmonary edema?**

A. A reduction in left atrial filling pressure or preload can be accomplished by several therapeutic interventions including sitting the patient upright, administering nitroglycerin, and administering diuretics.
B. The beneficial effect of morphine sulfate in this condition depends in part on a reduction in preload to the heart because morphine causes systemic venodilation.
C. Nitroprusside is a potent vasodilator for decreasing both systemic blood pressure and venous return.

D. Myocardial contractility can be augmented with dobutamine, an effect that may be associated with a decline in left atrial pressure.

Question 22.4. Which of the following statements regarding the potential beneficial effect of positive pressure ventilation and acute cardiogenic pulmonary edema is/are correct?

A. There may be an improvement in arterial oxygen saturation leading to better myocardial oxygen supply.
B. There may be a reduction in the extreme pleural pressure swings present with spontaneous ventilation, thus reducing afterload on the left ventricle.
C. There may be less workload on the failing heart because the work of breathing and the oxygen needed to perform it have been assumed by a mechanical ventilator.
D. There may be a reduction in atrial filling pressure or preload because positive pressure ventilation decreases venous return.

Question 22.5. Which of the following statements regarding the adult respiratory distress syndrome are true or false?

A. The primary mechanism of the arterial hypoxemia is due to right to left intrapulmonary shunting.
B. There is normally an increase in static lung compliance in patients with ARDS.
C. Bilateral infiltrates on the chest radiograph are required to make the diagnosis of acute lung injury or ARDS.
D. An important exclusion criterion for the diagnosis of acute lung injury or ARDS is the absence of clinical evidence for left ventricular failure or a pulmonary arterial wedge pressure greater than 18 mm Hg.

Question 22.6. Which of the following clinical disorders have been clearly associated with the development of acute lung injury or ARDS?

A. Inhaled toxins such as smoke or corrosive chemicals
B. Acute pancreatitis
C. Viral pneumonia
D. Trauma associated with fat emboli

Question 22.7. Which of the following statements regarding gastric aspiration are true or false?

A. The severity of lung injury is usually related inversely to the pH of the aspirated gastric contents.
B. Secondary bacterial lung infections play a minor role in the clinical course of lung injury from gastric aspiration.
C. Atelectasis may be an important part of the lung injury that occurs from aspiration of gastric contents.

Question 22.8. A 41-year-old gentleman developed Gram-negative sepsis that led to systemic hypotension, clinical evidence of septic shock, and the development of bilateral pulmonary infiltrates consistent with ARDS. Which of the following statements is/are correct about septic induced ARDS?

A. Pulmonary edema fluid that is aspirated from the endotracheal tube early in the course of ARDS from sepsis will normally have a protein concentration equal to approximately 80–100% of plasma protein concentration.
B. There is normally a reduction in the functional residual capacity of the lung because

edema fluid displaces air, thus decreasing gas volumes and also because there may be a reduction in functional surfactant in the alveoli.

C. Histologically, the lung typically shows acute inflammatory cells, red blood cells, and evidence of protein rich pulmonary edema.

D. Even though some patients with septic induced lung injury recover from the acute phase of severe pulmonary edema, their clinical course may be complicated by progressive fibrosing alveolitis and persistent respiratory failure.

Question 22.9. **Which of the following statements regarding mortality in patients with ARDS are true or false?**

A. Mortality is infrequently related to respiratory failure alone.
B. Sepsis is an important cause of mortality in ARDS only in the early phase of the syndrome.
C. Multiple organ failure is an important cause of the high mortality in patients with ARDS.

Question 22.10. **Which of the following statement regarding treatment for patients with ARDS is/are correct?**

A. Corticosteroids have no proven value in the treatment of ARDS.
B. However, antioxidant agents have been demonstrated to be of therapeutic value in treatment of ARDS.
C. Respiratory muscle fatigue is an uncommon clinical finding in patients with ARDS.
D. Mechanical ventilation with positive pressure is usually necessary to improve oxygenation and to stabilize alveolar ventilation in patients with ARDS.

Question 22.11. **Which of the following statements regarding the use of positive end expiratory pressure (PEEP) are true or false?**

A. PEEP does not alter the course of the primary lung injury.
B. However, PEEP may decrease extravascular lung water.
C. PEEP may also decrease cardiac output.
D. Use of PEEP usually allows the fraction of inspired oxygen tension to be reduced.

ANSWERS

Answer 22.1. **A, C**

The Starling equation indicates that an increase in hydrostatic pressure within any vascular space causes increased filtration. A decline in protein osmotic pressure will result in more filtration, not a rise in microvascular protein osmotic pressure. An increase in microvascular permeability is, of course, a common mechanism that results in increased movement of fluid across the vascular barrier. Lung lymphatics are important under normal as well as pathologic conditions for removing interstitial fluid from the lung.

Reference: pages 593–595

Answer 22.2. **A, B, D-True; C-False**

Interstitial and alveolar edema developed under conditions of hydrostatic stress in a progressive, stepwise fashion as left atrial pressure rises. Protein concentration is low in edema fluid because the microvascular barrier is not injured and therefore most of the filtered fluid has a low protein concentration. Pleural effusions form in the presence of pulmonary edema from movement of interstitial fluid across the visceral pleura into the pleural space.

Reference: pages 596–598

Answer 22.3.   All are correct

Several treatment modalities can decrease preload to the heart including a change in body position as well as pharmacologic therapy. Dobutamine, in contrast to dopamine, will lower left atrial pressure modestly while at the same time increasing myocardial contractility and modestly decreasing systemic vascular resistance.

Reference: pages 598–599

Answer 22.4.   All are correct

The beneficial effects of positive pressure ventilation and acute cardiogenic pulmonary edema are often overlooked. There is a good physiologic basis for the benefit of positive pressure ventilation in this clinical setting.

Reference: page 599

Answer 22.5.   A, C, D-True; B-False

These are all important characteristics of the adult respiratory distress syndrome except static lung compliance is normally decreased.

Reference: page 599

Answer 22.6.   All are correct

There are several clinical conditions that have been associated with the adult respiratory distress syndrome. See Table 22.2 for a comprehensive list.

Reference: page 601

Answer 22.7.   A, C-True; B-False

Aspiration of gastric contents is the second most common cause of acute lung injury in the adult respiratory distress syndrome (ARDS). The experimental studies indicate that anti-interleukin-8 (not anti-interleukin-b) therapy may be effective in preventing the severe pulmonary injury after acid aspiration. Secondary lung infections may play a major role in ARDS following aspiration induced lung injury.

Reference: pages 600–601

Answer 22.8.   All are correct

The clinical and pathologic findings in ARDS are similar regardless of the clinical disorder associated with ARDS. Even if patients do recover from the acute phase of severe pulmonary edema, they may still have a complicated course of severe respiratory failure secondary to fibrosing alveolitis, persistent respiratory failure, and an ongoing increased susceptibility to nosocomial infections.

Reference: page 602

Answer 22.9.   A, C-True; B-False

The most common cause of mortality in patients with ARDS is sepsis, both in the early and late phase of the syndrome. Non-pulmonary complications are an important major cause of a poor outcome in patients with ARDS.

Reference: page 604

Answer 22.10.   **D**

There are no pharmacologic agents that have been proven to be of treatment benefit in ARDS. Respiratory muscle fatigue may certainly occur in patients with ARDS, either in the early phase or in the later phase when they are being weaned from mechanical ventilation. More than 90% of patients with acute lung injury or ARDS will require positive pressure ventilation to treat their respiratory failure.

Reference: pages 604–605

Answer 22.11.   **A, C, D-True; B-False**

Positive end expiratory pressure (PEEP) is of value in improving oxygenation in patients with ARDS. It does allow a decrease in the fraction of inspired oxygen that needs to be used in most patients. However, it does not appear to have any direct effect on altering the course of lung injury or decreasing lung water. PEEP may also have adverse hemodynamic consequences such as decreasing cardiac output because of a decrease in venous return and preload to the heart.

Reference: page 605

chapter 23

Principles of Managing the Patient With Hemodynamic Insufficiency and Shock

QUESTIONS

Question 23.1. Which of the following statements regarding systemic arterial catheterization is/are correct?

A. Systemic arterial catheters are most useful for monitoring patients who are hemodynamically unstable.
B. Systemic arterial catheters are useful as a means for obtaining repeated blood samples from patients.
C. Systemic arterial catheters are usually well tolerated.
D. The most usually chosen site for insertion of a systemic arterial catheter is the brachial artery.

Question 23.2. Which of the following statements regarding complications of systemic arterial catheters are true or false?

A. Ischemia may occur most commonly secondary to thrombosis with local occlusion of the catheter.
B. The risk factors favoring infection include insertion by surgical cutdown rather than percutaneously and the duration of cannulation, particularly if it exceeds 4 days.
C. Continuous flush devices only increase the risk of infection.
D. The Allen's test is of little clinical utility.

Questions 23.3. Which of the following statements regarding insertion techniques for pulmonary arterial catheterization is/are correct?

A. Percutaneous insertion rather than a cutdown is usually adequate for inserting a pulmonary artery catheter into the pulmonary artery.
B. The proximal lumen on the pulmonary arterial catheter is normally located approximately 30 cm from the tip of the catheter and when appropriately positioned in the right atrium this proximal lumen will provide a measurement of central venous pressure.
C. This same proximal lumen is ordinarily used to inject a bolus of indicator (usually 10 mL of 5% dextrose saline) to determine cardiac output by thermodilution.
D. Cardiac output is determined by bedside computer that integrates the time/temperature curve and prints out the cardiac output.

Question 23.4. Which of the following statements are True or False regarding measurement of pressures with a pulmonary arterial catheter?

A. Pulmonary arterial pressure measurements in and of themselves do not depend on calibrated transducers.

B. Correct amplitude settings are necessary to display the pressure waveforms on the bedside oscilloscope.
C. The effects of respiration on measuring central venous or pulmonary arterial wedge pressure measurements are only critical if the patient is being mechanically ventilated with positive pressure.
D. Ideally, measurements of pulmonary arterial wedge pressure should be made at the end of expiration.

Question 23.5. Which of the following statements is/are correct regarding accurate measurements of pulmonary arterial pressure?

A. Measurement of pulmonary arterial pressures including pulmonary arterial wedge pressure is often difficult in patients with severe airway obstruction.
B. During inspiration, the patient's pleural pressure may be negative if he or she is spontaneously breathing.
C. It is important to note the period of end expiration, whether the patient is spontaneously breathing or being ventilated with positive pressure.
D. The correlation between pulmonary arterial wedge pressure and left atrial pressure is generally quite good.

Question 23.6. Which of the following statements are True or False regarding the relationship of positive-end expiratory pressure to the measurement of pulmonary arterial wedge pressure?

A. PEEP has no effect on pulmonary arterial wedge pressure if the measurement is made at the end of expiration.
B. Esophageal pressure can be measured to provide an index of pleural pressure in patients being treated with PEEP.
C. The transmission of PEEP to the pleural space is uncertain and depends in part on the compliance of the lungs.
D. In order to determine if the tip of the catheter is in a zone 3 location, several maneuvers can be taken to assess this issue.

Question 23.7. Which of the following are reasonable clinical indications for catheterization of patients?

A. Acute cardiac insufficiency in a medical or surgical patient in which vasodilator or vasopressor therapy might be used.
B. To distinguish cardiogenic from noncardiogenic pulmonary edema.
C. To determine the etiology of shock.
D. To guide the management of patients undergoing major vascular surgery who have a history of ischemic cardiac disease.

Question 23.8. Which of the following statements regarding the physiologic basis for shock are True or False?

A. The diagnosis of shock does not depend on a specific level of systolic blood pressure as much as it does on evidence of end organ hypoperfusion.
B. Peripheral vasodilatation is characteristic of septic shock whereas vasoconstriction occurs most commonly in cardiogenic and hypovolemic shock.
C. Determination of optimal left ventricular preload is important in all types of shock.
D. It is rare for a patient to have two mechanisms to account for their shock.

ANSWERS

Answer 23.1.   **A, B, C**

Systemic arterial catheters are very useful and important in monitoring critically ill patients. They are normally inserted, however, in the radial artery, although occasionally in the femoral artery.

Reference: pages 609–610

Answer 23.2.   **A, B-True; C, D-False**

The use of a continuous flush device located immediately distal to the transducer rather than close to the insertion site has proved to be helpful in reducing catheter-related infection in systemic arterial catheters. Secondly, an Allen's test can be of significant clinical value. Ulnar refill time is determined by the Allen's test prior to the insertion of a catheter in the radial artery. A Palmar blush should occur from filling of the distal hand by blood from the ulnar artery within 5 seconds of occluding flow through the radial artery.

Reference: page 610

Answer 23.3.   **All are correct**

Reference: pages 610, 611

Answer 23.4.   **B, D-True; A, C-False**

Correct calibration of transducers is needed to obtain correct pressure measurements. In general, amplitudes in the range of 0–60 mm Hg are appropriate for the pulmonary circulation. Changes in pleural pressure with respiration can affect pressure measurements whether the patient is spontaneously breathing or being ventilated with positive pressure. In any case, all pressure measurements should be made at the end of expiration when pleural pressure is likely to be nearest zero.

Reference: pages 611, 612

Answer 23.5.   **All are correct**

Acute airway obstruction makes it difficult to measure pulmonary arterial pressures accurately because of the rapid swings in pleural pressure. Measurement of pressures at the end of expiration is critical to obtaining accurate transmural pressures. In general, the relationship between pulmonary arterial wedge pressure and left atrial pressure is good, provided that the tip of the pulmonary arterial catheter is in a zone 3 area of the lung.

Reference: pages 613, 614

Answer 23.6.   **B, C, D-True; A-False**

PEEP may influence the measured arterial wedge pressure because it may result in a rise in pleural pressure or pressure surrounding vascular bed, thus resulting in a lower transmural pressure measurement than is actually reflected in the intraluminal measurement alone. Although esophageal pressure can be measured, it is not routinely available in critically ill patients and it is a difficult measurement to do accurately in the supine patient. The fraction of PEEP that is transmitted to the pleural space is uncertain, particularly in the presence of acute and chronic lung disease. Table 23.1 on page 615 lists several of the maneuvers that can be done to verify the position of the pulmonary arterial catheter in a zone 3 area of the lung.

Reference: pages 614, 615

Answer 23.7.   **All are correct**

Although there is some uncertainty regarding the absolute indication for pulmonary arterial catheterization in critically ill patients, it is generally true that patients with a history of cardiac disease are the most likely patients to benefit from pulmonary arterial catheterization. The reason for this conclusion is that there is effective pharmacologic therapy that can be used in patients with cardiac dysfunction to alter the course of their disease. In contrast, in patients with ARDS, the utility of measuring pulmonary arterial wedge pressure is usually limited to determining whether the patient has unexpected cardiac rather than noncardiac pulmonary edema. In a few patients with ARDS, a modestly elevated pulmonary arterial wedge pressure may indicate that diuretic therapy could be helpful, but the fundamental disease process is not affected by pulmonary arterial catheterization.

Reference: pages 615, 616

Answer 23.8.   **A, B, C-True; D-False**

Shock is best defined by hypoperfusion of end organs as reflected clinically by a decrease in mental status, oliguria, cold, clammy skin, and other indices of poor tissue perfusion. Vasodilatation is more characteristic of septic shock. In patient with sepsis, typically the cardiac output is increased rather than decreased. Finally, it is not uncommon for patients to have two mechanisms for their shock. For example, septic shock may be complicated by significant intravascular volume depletion. Also, cardiogenic shock may be complicated by hypovolemia. See Table 23.2 for further details.

Reference: pages 615–617

chapter 24

Sepsis and Multiple Organ Failure

QUESTIONS

Question 24.1. **Which of the following statements regarding the definition and epidemiology of multiple organ failure is/are correct?**

A. Multiple organ failure is often a major complication in patients from shock of almost any etiology.
B. The organ dysfunction that may occur is variable from patients and not easily predictable.
C. Cardiovascular failure among critically ill patients varies from 10–25%.
D. Renal failure does not occur in the absence of acute respiratory failure.

Question 24.2. **Which of the following statements are true or false regarding acute renal failure?**

A. Nephrotoxic drugs are a common cause of oliguric renal failure.
B. Hypotension from sepsis or other causes may result in acute renal failure.
C. Nonoliguric renal failure has a better prognosis than oliguric renal failure.

Question 24.3. **In reference to gastrointestinal and hepatic failure in critically ill patients, which of the following statements is/are correct?**

A. Clinical features of gastric tract dysfunction may include hemorrhage, ileus, acalculous cholecystitis, or pancreatitis.
B. Interruption of the mucosal integrity of the gastrointestinal tract may lead to translocation of bacteria into the peritoneal cavity or regional gastrointestinal lymph nodes.
C. A reversible elevation in liver function tests is common in critically ill patients.
D. Significant liver dysfunction is indicated by an elevation in bilirubin to 4–5 mg/dL, an increase in the prothrombin time of more than 1.5 times control, and a serum albumin below 2.5 g/dL.

Question 24.4. **In regard to central nervous system failure in critically ill patients, which of the following statements are true or false?**

A. Sepsis can be associated with a decrease in mental alertness and overall mental status without focal findings in as many as 30–35% of patients.
B. The Glasgow Coma Scale provides a measurement of visual, motor, and verbal responsiveness that can be quantified.
C. The factors that lead to central nervous system dysfunction in critically ill patients may include the production of false neurotransmitters, direct microvascular injury, and even brain ischemia.

Question 24.5. **A 45-year-old patient was admitted to the intensive care unit with the diagnosis of ARDS. He had a chest radiograph that showed bilateral dense pul-**

monary infiltrates in all four quadrants. His arterial oxygen tension was 60 mm Hg on an FiO_2 of 0.8. He was mechanically ventilated with positive pressure ventilation. His tidal volume was 1000 mL with a plateau pressure of 50 cm H_2O with a positive-end expiratory pressure of 10 cm H_2O. Which of the following statements regarding his acute lung injury score is/are correct?

A. The patient should be assigned 4 points for his abnormalities on chest radiograph.
B. The patient should be assigned 4 points for his hypoxemia score.
C. The patient should be assigned 3 points for his respiratory system compliance score.
D. The patient should be assigned 4 points for his PEEP score.

ANSWERS

Answer 24.1. **A, B, C-True; D-False**

Acute renal failure may occur as a single complication of shock but may also occur in association with other organ failure such as hepatic or respiratory failure.

Reference: pages 619–620

Answer 24.2. **B, C-True; A-False**

Nephrotoxic renal failure (most commonly from aminoglycoside antibiotic therapy) usually causes non-oliguric renal failure.

Reference: page 620

Answer 24.3. **A, B, C, D are correct**

Liver dysfunction is a major complication in critically ill patients, especially when it is severe. The basic mechanisms of liver injury in critically ill patients, however, are not well worked out.

Reference: page 621

Answer 24.4. **A, B, C-True**

Details of the Glasgow Coma Scale are provided in Table 24.1.

Reference: page 621

Answer 24.5. **A, B, C are correct**

The first three statements are true but the PEEP score should be 2 since his PEEP level was 10 cm H_2O. See Table 24.2 for the components of the acute lung injury score. This patient's total score was greater than 2.5 when the aggregate sum is divided by the four components that were used. This would place him in the category of severe acute lung injury category.

Reference: page 622

chapter 25

Thoracic Trauma, Surgery and Perioperative Management

QUESTIONS

Question 25.1. **Regarding the effects of general anesthesia on pulmonary physiology, which of the following statements is/are correct?**

A. Pulmonary gas exchange may be impaired during general anesthesia and can result in intraoperative and postoperative hypoxemia.
B. Approximately a 20% reduction in functional residual capacity typically occurs in patients who assume the supine position, even independent of muscular paralysis.
C. Obesity may worsen the decline of functional residual capacity that occurs with assuming the supine position.
D. A further reduction of functional residual capacity may occur with the induction of general anesthesia and muscle relaxation, and patients with elevated closing capacities will be the more predisposed to atelectasis with the induction of general anesthesia.

Question 25.2. **Which of the following statements regarding the use of postoperative epidural analgesia are true or false?**

A. Postoperative epidural analgesia may provide good pain relief.
B. Postoperative epidural analgesia reduces postoperative respiratory complications.
C. Postoperative respiratory depression may occur with the use of epidural morphine.
D. Systemic hypotension may also be associated with the use of epidural analgesia.

Question 25.3. **Which of the following are risk factors for postoperative atelectasis?**

A. Upper abdominal surgery.
B. History of smoking.
C. Obesity.
D. Age greater than 50 years old.

Question 25.4. **Which of the following statements are true or false regarding the cardiorespiratory effects of smoking?**

A. Smoking decreases myocardial oxygen consumption.
B. Smoking may cause coronary artery vasospasm.
C. Smoking may shift the oxyhemoglobin association curve to the right.
D. Smoking decreases mucociliary clearance from the lung.

Question 25.5. **Which of the following statements is/are correct regarding preoperative measures that can reduce the incidence of postoperative pulmonary complications in patients with COPD?**

A. There is no evidence that cessation of smoking preoperatively will reduce postoperative complications.
B. Treatment with inhaled bronchodilators preoperatively may reduce the incidence of postoperative complications.
C. All antibiotics regardless of whether the patients sputum is purulent may reduce the incidence of postoperative pulmonary complications.
D. A preoperative exercise program has been shown to reduce postoperative pulmonary complications and COPD.

Question 25.6.   **A 48-year-old gentleman with a life-long history of moderate to severe asthma is scheduled to undergo elective surgery for a cholecystectomy. He will be intubated and ventilated for this procedure. Which of the following anesthetic maneuvers may precipitate bronchospasm in this patient?**

A. Direct airway irritation by tracheal intubation.
B. Ventilation of cool, dry gases.
C. The administration of intravenous morphine can cause histamine release.
D. Use of a neuromuscular blocking agents such as atracurium.

Question 25.7.   **Which of the following statements are true or false regarding the effects of obesity on pulmonary function?**

A. These patients have a decrease in chest wall compliance.
B. The decrease in chest wall compliance can reduce lung volume and lead to an increase in work of breathing.
C. Patients with obesity may have a reduction in functional residual capacity which may predispose to early airway closure.
D. There may be a widened alveolar-oxygen gradient in obese patients at baseline simply because of their low closing volume and early airway closure.

Question 25.8.   **Which of the following statements regarding preoperative factors related to postoperative cardiac complications is/are correct?**

A. The presence of either an S_3 gallop or jugular venous distention.
B. Myocardial infarction within the past 2 years.
C. Any cardiac rhythm other than sinus.
D. Age over 60 years.

Question 25.9.   **Which of the following statements is/are correct regarding preoperative work-up for assessment of whether a patient can tolerate lung resection?**

A. Arresting arterial $PCO_2 > 45$ mm Hg usually means the patient should not undergo resectional surgery.
B. A patient with greater than 50% of predicted pulmonary function following lung resection should be allowed to undergo surgery.
C. Perfusion lung scan is helpful in evaluating patients for resectional lung surgery, particularly if the predicted postoperative pulmonary function is less than 50% of predicted.
D. Exercise testing provides an additional important evaluation test in patient who have borderline predicted postoperative pulmonary function following lung resection surgery.

Question 25.10.   **Which of the following statements are true or false regarding the risk of complications in nonresectional surgery?**

A. There is little evidence of benefit of pulmonary function testing as a routine screening technique in the absence of clinical symptoms.
B. Patients with chronic obstructive lung disease often have an increased incidence of postoperative pulmonary complications following abdominal surgery.
C. Patients who undergo abdominal vascular surgery have been shown to have an increased risk of postoperative respiratory failure and the need for mechanical ventilation if they have a long history of cigarette smoking, preoperative hypoxemia, as well as a significant intraoperative blood loss.
D. Postponing surgery is more important for procedures in the upper abdomen than for other procedures.

Question 25.11. Nosocomial pneumonia occurs most frequently in surgical patients and it is the third most frequent cause of nosocomial infection after urinary tract infections and wound infections. Postoperative nosocomial pneumonia also has a mortality rate that approaches 50%. Which of the following factors increase the risk of postoperative pneumonia?

A. Increased length of preoperative and hospital stay.
B. Atelectasis.
C. Emergency operation.
D. Severe underlying illness such as peritonitis, sepsis, or burn.

Question 25.12. Which of the following statements regarding aspiration of gastric contents are true or false?

A. Patients with gastric and small bowel obstruction have increased gastric volume which may increase intragastric pressure and increase the risk for aspiration of gastric contents.
B. Patients may not recover normal glottic closure for up to eight hours after extubation.
C. If intubated, patients cannot aspirate oral pharyngeal contents.
D. The severity of aspiration lung injury is greater if the pH is less than 2.5 or the volume is greater than 25 ml.

Question 25.13. Which of the following statements regarding thoracic trauma is/are correct?

A. Thoracic injuries are directly responsible for 25% of all nonmilitary deaths in the United States.
B. Patients with thoracic trauma frequently have coexisting extrathoracic injuries; however, the thoracic components of the injury are the ones that pose the greatest threat to survival in the first few hours.
C. Potentially life-threatening injuries must be identified rapidly in the emergency room with a detailed head to toe physical exam.
D. Volume resuscitation takes precedence over airway management.

Question 25.14. A 41-year-old man is admitted to the intensive care unit following thoracic trauma. He has evidence of a flail chest. Which of the following statements are true or false regarding flail chest injuries?

A. Pulmonary function abnormalities observed in flail chest injuries include a decrease in vital capacity, an increase in functional residual capacity, and a decrease in airway resistance.
B. Current guidelines for management of flail chest injuries to the chest recommend

volume ventilation if the respiratory rate is over 40 or there is a progressive decrease in vital capacity to less than 10 ml/kg body weight or there is hypercapnia.

C. The criteria for extubation of a patient with a flail chest injury are more stringent than patients without a flail chest injury.

D. There is evidence of long-term pulmonary disability in patients who have had a flail chest injury.

Question 25.15. Which of the following statements regarding hemothorax is/are correct?

A. Initial treatment of any large hemothorax is the evacuation of the pleural cavity with a large bore chest tube.

B. Shock may be the presenting feature of massive hemothorax.

C. As much as 1 liter of blood can occupy one hemothorax.

D. Auto transfusion devices should not be used to reinfuse blood from a patient who has a traumatic hemothorax.

Question 25.16. A 52-year-old woman is admitted to the intensive care unit following severe trauma from a motor vehicle accident in which she sustained several local extremity long bone fractures as well as a pelvic fracture. She is at high risk for fat embolism syndrome. Which of the following constitute major criteria for the diagnosis of fat embolism syndrome?

A. Hypoxemia, PaO_2 <60 mm Hg on an FiO_2 of 0.40

B. Pulmonary edema

C. CNS depression

D. Axillary or conjunctival petechiae

Question 25.17. Which of the following statements regarding esophageal perforation are true or false?

A. Perforation of rupture of the esophagus can occur spontaneously or following trauma, instrumentation, or foreign body ingestion.

B. The diagnosis of perforation of the esophagus may be difficult.

C. Spontaneous perforation can occur with forceful emesis.

D. The most dreaded complication of esophageal perforation is mediastinal sepsis.

ANSWERS

Answer 25.1. **A, B, C, D are correct**

All of these statements are correct and indicate that the supine position accompanied with general anesthesia and muscle paralysis predisposes to atelectasis and postoperative hypoxemia, especially because the normal pulmonary hypoxic vasoconstrictor response may be blunted by the use of inhalation anesthetics.

Reference: page 630

Answer 25.2. **A, C, D-True; B-False**

There is no clear evidence that epidural analgesia decreases the instance of postoperative respiratory complications. However, it definitely has excellent analgesic properties and reduces the need for systemic narcotics. Uncommonly, respiratory depression or systemic hypotension may occur, thus careful patient monitoring is important.

Reference: page 631

Answer 25.3.   **A, B, C are correct**

The first three factors (upper abdominal surgery, smoking, and postoperative immobility) are all significant risk factors for postoperative atelectasis. Age greater than 70, not age greater than 50, is an established risk factor also; therefore, statement 4 is incorrect. Other postoperative risk factors for atelectasis are a thoracotomy, bypass surgery with external cardiac hypothermia, chronic obstructive pulmonary disease, restrictive pulmonary disease, and obesity. Please see Table 25.2.

Reference: page 631

Answer 25.4.   **B, D-True; A, C-False**

Smoking can have several undesirable effects on cardiac and respiratory function. Smoking can decrease resistance to infection by decreasing neutrophil chemotaxis, decreasing circulating immunoglobulin levels, decreasing pulmonary macrophage count, and other immune suppressant effects. See Table 25.3.

Reference: page 633

Answer 25.5.   **B, D are correct**

Although there is some disagreement among studies that have been done, one classic study reported that pulmonary complications in patients with COPD can be reduced approximately 2- to 3-fold with a preoperative pulmonary preparation program consisting of cessation of smoking, treatment of inhaled bronchodilators, and oral antibiotics if the sputum is purulent.

Reference: page 633

Answer 25.6.   **A, B, C, D are correct**

The first three statements are correct but the last statement is not correct. Use of neuromuscular blockers in the operating room does not precipitate bronchospasm although there is some old literature that suggests this could happen with curare because of its potential to release histamine. Curare is infrequently used in clinical practice now.

Reference: page 634

Answer 25.7.   **A, B, C, D are correct**

All the above statements regarding the impact of obesity on pulmonary function are correct. In addition, obesity imposes a stress on the cardiovascular system with an increase in circulating blood volume and increased metabolic demand.

Reference: page 635

Answer 25.8.   **A, C are correct**

There are several well identified preoperative factors that are related to postoperative cardiac complications. Statements 1 and 3 are true. However, myocardial infarction in the past six months, not the last two years, is an important risk factor. Also, age over 70 years, not over 60 years, is an important risk factor. Other important risk factors include more than five documented premature ventricular contractions per minute, intraperitoneal, intrathoracic, or an aortic operation, clinically significant aortic stenosis, poor general medical condition, and emergency operation. Please see Table 25.4.

Reference: page 635

Answer 25.9.   A, B, C, D are correct

Not infrequently, a potential candidate for lung resectional surgery will fall into a borderline category in which the predicted FEV_1 is in the range of 0.8 to 1 liter. Noninvasive cardiopulmonary exercise testing appears to be an excellent approach to evaluating these patients. If their maximum oxygen consumption is less than 10 ml/minute/kg, then most authorities recommend no surgery.

Reference: pages 637–638

Answer 25.10.   A, B, C, D-True

More studies are needed to understand the specific factors that can predict postoperative pulmonary complications in subgroups. It is clear, however, that abdominal surgery is a major risk in patients with obstructive lung disease although preoperative pulmonary function tests do not accurately predict which patients will develop postoperative respiratory failure.

Reference: pages 637–639

Answer 25.11.   A, B, C, D are correct

There are several factors that increase the risk for postoperative pneumonia. All of the above-listed factors are identified risk factors. Other factors include emergency operation, prolonged operation, history of smoking, malnutrition, history of aspiration, and obesity. See Table 25.5.

Reference: page 640

Answer 25.12.   A, B, D-True; C-False

All of the above statements are true regarding aspiration of gastric contents except statement C. Note that mortality from significant gastric aspiration can be as high as 10–30%. Please see Chapter 22 for a discussion of ARDS resulting from aspiration of gastric contents.

Reference: pages 640–641

Answer 25.13.   A, B, C are correct

Initial management of treatment must include the ABCs, which means management of airway, breathing, and circulation. So management of the airway is primary and coexistent with management of circulatory insufficiency. The primary and secondary survey of immediately and potentially life-threatening injuries must be done rapidly and comprehensively (see Table 25.7).

Reference: page 642

Answer 25.14.   B, C, D-True; A-False

The first statement is not correct because pulmonary function abnormalities in flail chest injury result in a decrease in vital capacity and a decrease in residual capacity, not an increase in functional residual capacity. Also, there is typically an increase in airway resistance and the work of breathing. The other statements are true.

Reference: pages 644–645

Answer 25.15.   A, B, C

Auto transfusion devices can be used for infusion of shed blood from hemothorax. Up to 5 liters of blood may be retransfused in this fashion without any documented ill effects. The need for exploratory thoracotomy generally depends on the rate of bleeding.

Reference: page 646

Answer 25.16.   A, B, C, D are correct

The diagnosis of fat embolism syndrome can be difficult since the findings are common in many patients, although the combination of the above four findings in the right clinical setting makes the diagnosis very likely. Clinical presentation of fat embolism syndrome typically begins with pulmonary signs of dyspnea, tachypnea, and respiratory distress as early as 4 hours following trauma or major orthopedic surgery. Central nervous system disturbances occur about this time and range from mild disorientation to seizures and coma. The development of petechiae is typically delayed by several hours and found later on the chest, axillae, groin, or conjunctivae.

Reference: page 648

Answer 25.17.   A, B, C, D-True

As stated above, the diagnosis of esophageal perforation can be difficult because symptoms may initially be absent. Examination may reveal subcutaneous emphysema and a mediastinal crunch may be heard on auscultation. On chest radiograph, a wide mediastinum may be present. Management usually involves surgery, but nonoperative treatment may be effective.

Reference: pages 653–654.

chapter 26

Metabolism, Nutrition, and Respiration in Critically Ill Patients

QUESTIONS

Question 26.1. **Which of the following statements regarding nutritional support in the critically ill patient is/are correct?**

A. There is evidence that optimal early nutritional will decrease the rate of infection.
B. There is evidence that early nutritional support may improve wound healing.
C. There is evidence that nutritional support may maintain the integrity of the gastrointestinal tract, particularly decreasing bacterial translocation.
D. There is evidence that enteral feeding is preferable to parenteral nutrition.

Question 26.2. **Which of the following statements are true or false regarding fuel utilization during critical illness?**

A. Oxidative metabolism of fat yields considerably more energy than that of protein or glucose.
B. During the initial phase of nonstress starvation (a few days), glycogen stores are broken down to provide the glucose necessary for the brain, red blood cells, white blood cells, and kidneys.
C. Nonstress starvation normally leads to death in approximately 2 months.

Question 26.3. **Patients with burns, trauma, or sepsis, protein catabolism markedly exceeds protein synthesis. Which of the following statements is/are correct regarding protein metabolism during these illnesses?**

A. Thirty grams of muscle mass contains 6.25 g of protein, which when fully catabolized leads to 1 g of urinary nitrogen excretion.
B. Daily urinary nitrogen excretion may range from 20–30 g with trauma or sepsis.
C. These major losses can lead to life threatening protein malnutrition within 1–2 weeks.
D. Amino acids produced in the breakdown of protein are used to produce glucose and acute phase reactant proteins.

Question 26.4. **Which of the following statements regarding nutritional assessment in critically ill patients is/are correct?**

A. A serum albumin of less than 2.4 g/dL suggests severe protein deficiency but may also be low because of other clinical problems including fluid overload, congestive heart failure, or liver failure.
B. Transferrin has a half-life of 9 days and is usually decreased in malnutrition, but it may be normal in iron deficiency and it may be decreased simply because of fluid overload and stress.

C. Anthropometric measurements have limited usefulness in critically ill patients because they cannot detect acute changes.
D. Measurement of plasma prealbumin is very sensitive, however, to malnutrition in critically ill patients.

Question 26.5. Which of the following statements regarding estimation of energy requirements are true or false?

A. Basal resting energy expenditure may be estimated from the Harris-Benidick equation which depends on the patient's gender, weight, height, and age.
B. Indirect calorimetry measures oxygen consumption and carbon dioxide production.
C. The respiratory quotient is defined as the ratio of oxygen uptake to carbon dioxide production.
D. Indirect calorimetry is difficult to do in patients who are being treated with a fraction of inspired oxygen concentration above 0.5.

Question 26.6. Which of the following statements is/are correct regarding nitrogen requirements?

A. Nitrogen is excreted via the kidneys, the skin, and the gut.
B. Each gram of urinary nitrogen results in the breakdown of 6.25 grams of protein (equivalent to approximately to 30 g of muscle mass).
C. In critically ill patients, 30–40 g of urinary nitrogen may be encountered.
D. The patient's nitrogen balance is determined by calculating protein intake divided by 6.25—urinary losses plus 4 g for gastrointestinal losses.

Question 26.7. Which of the following are common causes of diarrhea in critically ill patients?

A. *Clostridium difficile*
B. Hypertonic feeding solutions
C. Antibiotics
D. Magnesium-containing antacids

Question 26.8. Which of the following nutrients are particularly important for enteral alimentation?

A. Glutamine
B. Vitamin B_{12}
C. Arginine
D. Epidermal growth factor

Question 26.9. Which of the following statements regarding the potential advantages of enteral versus parenteral nutrition are true or false?

A. Enteral nutrition is cheaper than parenteral nutrition.
B. Enteral nutrition is easier and less invasive to administer than parenteral nutrition.
C. Enteral nutrition appears to maintain the immune function of the gut.
D. Enteral nutrition does contain some nutrients such as complex carbohydrates, fiber, and glutamine that are not contained in total parenteral nutritional fluids.

Question 26.10. Which of the following statements is/are correct regarding respiratory complications that may occur when refeeding is initiated in malnourished patients?

A. There will be increased ventilatory demands from the secondary increase in carbon dioxide production.

B. Electrolyte abnormalities such as hypophosphatemia may occur.
C. Hypokalemia may result, which can cause clinically significant muscle weakness.
D. Hypomagnesemia may also occur with a resultant decrease in muscle strength and possibly a decrease in effective alveolar ventilation.

ANSWERS

Answer 26.1. **A, B, C, D are correct**

Although guidelines for nutritional therapy in critically ill patients are not always based on rigorous, controlled studies, the above statements are true.

Reference: page 658

Answer 26.2. **A, B, C-True**

See Table 26.1 for specific details of the effects of nonstress starvation compared to hypermetabolic hypercatabolic stress.

Reference: page 659

Answer 26.3. **A, B, C, D are correct**

The rate of protein breakdown varies from patient to patient, but these are broad guidelines for the expected losses in severely ill patients.

Reference: pages 662–663

Answer 26.4. **A, B, C are correct**

All of the visceral proteins (Table 26.4) change too slowly to indicate either current nutritional status or acute changes in nutritional status with changes in therapy. Nutritional assessment in critically ill patients, therefore, must take into account specific aspects of the history including recent weight and recent caloric intake as well as estimated requirements, which may be increased because of infection. Also, physical examination is important to look for evidence of muscle wasting, fat loss, and peripheral edema.

Reference: pages 662–663

Answer 26.5. **A, B, D-True; C-False**

Statement D is false because the definition of respiratory quotient (RQ) is the ratio of carbon dioxide production to oxygen uptake. Although indirect calorimetry can be done, there is no evidence that use of the equipment to calculate this information alters patient outcome.

Reference: pages 664–665

Answer 26.6. **A, B, C, D are correct**

In patients with unstable renal function, the urinary nitrogen will not equal the protein breakdown. In this case, the change in total body BUN in grams has to be included so the nitrogen balance equation needs to be adjusted (see page 666). Note that with a negative nitrogen balance, normally one concludes that there is net protein loss. With proper nutritional replacement, the goal is to achieve and maintain a positive nitrogen balance.

Reference: page 665

Answer 26.7. **A, B, C, D are correct**

All of the above are causes of diarrhea particularly in critically ill patients. Other drugs that cause diarrhea, especially in critically ill patients, include H_2-receptor antagonists, metoclopramide, and sorbitol-containing theophylline elixirs. Bacterial overgrowth, protein calorie malnutrition, and decreased plasma protein concentration may also cause diarrhea.

Reference: page 667

Answer 26.8. **A, C are correct**

See the discussion on page 668 for further details.

Reference: page 668

Answer 26.9. **A, B, C, D-True**

There are several advantages of enteral over parenteral nutrition. However, controlled studies in patients have not been done that conclusively prove the superiority of enteral nutrition over parenteral nutrition in large numbers of patients with major outcome variables. Nevertheless, enteral nutrition has some obvious advantages.

Reference: page 669

Answer 26 10. **A, B, C, D are correct**

Please see Table 26.9 for other details. Ethical considerations must be considered in providing nutritional support.

Reference: pages 673–674

8:00 Am

5 & S

Rm411   1 + 3

Thurs